UNIVERSITY OF RHODE ISLAND LIBRARY

HEALTHY COMPANIES
A Human Resources Approach

Robert H. Rosen, Ph.D.

AMA Management Briefing

NO LONGER THE PROPERTY
OF THE
UNIVERSITY OF R. I. LIBRARY

AMA MEMBERSHIP PUBLICATIONS DIVISION
AMERICAN MANAGEMENT ASSOCIATION

Library of Congress Cataloging-in-Publication Data

Rosen, Robert H.
  Healthy companies.

  (AMA management briefing)
  1. Industrial hygiene. 2. Health promotion. I. Title.
II. Series.
RC967.R68   1986   613.6'2   86-22255
ISBN 0-8144-2329-9

©1986 Robert H. Rosen

All rights reserved. Printed in the United States of America.
This Management Briefing has been distributed to all members enrolled in the Human Resources Limited Company, and Insurance and Employee Benefits divisions of the American Management Association. Copies may be purchased at the following single-copy rates: AMA members, $7.50. Nonmembers, $10.00. Students, $3.75 (upon presentation of a college/university identification card at an AMA bookstore). Faculty members may purchase 25 or more copies for classroom use at the student discount rate (order on college letterhead).

This publication may not be reproduced, stored in a retrieval system, or transmitted in whole or in part, in any form or by any means, electronic, mechanical, photocopying, recording, or otherwise, without the prior written permission of AMA Membership Publications Division, 135 West 50th Street, New York, N.Y. 10020.

First Printing

About the Author

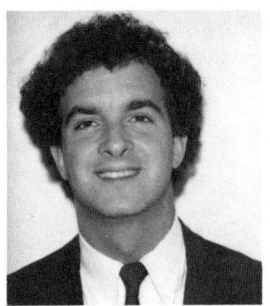

Robert H. Rosen is a clinical psychologist active in the national arena in areas of organizational health and worksite health enhancement. He promotes the concept of the "healthy corporation," and his primary interests revolve around the integration of training, organizational development, corporate culture, mental wellness, health promotion, management strategy, and health care cost management. In addition to writing numerous articles on organizational health, Dr. Rosen speaks nationally at conferences on healthy companies.

Dr. Rosen serves as consultant to the Washington Business Group on Health (WBGH), a membership organization of approximately 200 of the *Fortune* 500 companies and the only national organization devoted exclusively to the health and human resource policy and cost management needs of major employers. In his capacity as consultant to the WBGH, Dr. Rosen directs the Institute on Organizational Health and is also founding editor of *Corporate Commentary*, a national quarterly report on the evaluation of worksite health strategies. He has consulted to numerous private- and public-sector organizations, unions, and government-sponsored projects on organizational health, health promotion, and disease prevention. He also works with entrepreneur/owners of small businesses, assisting on various human resource issues.

Dr. Rosen is Assistant Clinical Professor of Psychiatry and Behavioral Sciences at the George Washington University School of Medicine. He received his Ph.D. at the University of Pittsburgh and completed postdoctoral work in the Department of Psychiatry at George Washington University and the Children's Hospital National Medical Center. Currently, Dr. Rosen is working on a new book entitled *The Healthy Corporation*, to be published by John Wiley in 1987.

Acknowledgments

This monograph is dedicated to a very special group of friends and colleagues whose diverse visions and backgrounds have guided and challenged me over the past five years to look beyond current ways of thinking and to examine new opportunities for nurturing and managing people inside organizations. I wish to express my sincere appreciation to Willis Goldbeck, Anne Kiefhaber, Ruth Behrens, Gail Ducrest, Jay Fisette, Stan Berlinsky, and Suzanne Goldberg for this support.

My deepest thanks go to Carol Freedman, my colleague and research associate, for her continued insights and commitment to what is possible.

Finally, my warmest regards go to Don Bohl and Anne Skagen of the American Management Association for their patience and faith in this work.

Contents

Introduction   9

Part I: What Is the Healthy Company?   15

1 Key Considerations of the "Healthy Corporation"   17
2 Trends Affecting Companies   22
3 Principles of Healthy Companies   29

Part II: Diagnosing Corporate Culture   33

4 Stressful Work Conditions   35
5 Lack of Control/Participation   48
6 Tense Work Relationships   60
7 Lack of Career Progress   71
8 Unclear Work Roles   77
9 Poorly Managed Change   82
10 Work/Family/Leisure Conflicts   90
11 Retirement   98

Appendix   103

Introduction

Historically, companies have tried a number of approaches to maximize the health and performance of their workforce. By offering health benefits and through their human resource policies, companies have tried to keep employees healthy and productive on the job. It is now part of conventional wisdom that healthy people produce better results. It's clear, however, that some companies are making better investments in human capital than others.

The healthy corporation differs dramatically from its unhealthy counterpart. The most profound difference is that the former promotes health and productivity together. In these companies, "peak performers" and "stress-resistant" employees are viewed as corporate assets, and the company does all it can to maximize their physical and mental health. Health care benefits and wellness programs are created to promote employee health, and work conditions and management policies are designed to support that end.

In contrast, unhealthy companies ignore the connection between health and productivity, and, in fact, often contribute to unhealthy stress and sickness in their employees. The result is unnecessary health and human resource costs, and reduced profits.

There are four major "health and productivity" divisions within a company: health benefits, occupational safety and health, prevention and wellness, and human resource development. Each makes a separate contribution toward promoting individual health and organizational profitability.

Unfortunately, one of the greatest barriers impeding both healthy and unhealthy companies today is that most approach health and productivity issues across several different departments, with little attempt to integrate their programs; indeed, a recently completed research effort identified twenty-six different corporate functions that related to the health of employees. Each department or "program area" has its own history, mission, language, responsibility, and professional identity, and in each the focus is either on health or productivity. Rarely are the two functions connected.

For example, in the health area, the benefits, safety, and employee assistance departments rule. In the areas of performance and productivity, departments like training, organizational development, and personnel relations head the list. Few departments are aware of the efforts of the others or of the potential for cooperation.

To illustrate this point, the four major health and productivity departments in most companies are discussed below.

HEALTH BENEFITS

As early as the 1930s, Blue Cross/Blue Shield and the commercial insurance carriers began offering insurance to the public to help make health care services more affordable. Since then, employers' responsibility for the health of employees and their families has increased markedly, and today most employers offer some type of health care benefits to their workers. Health care benefits have expanded to include major medical and hospitalization services, prescription drugs, dental care, care for drug abuse and alcoholism, vision care, podiatric services, home health services, and more recently hospice care and the use of birthing centers. Many companies have expanded their coverage to dependents.

Most large employers now also pick up the cost of health insurance for retirees to supplement Medicare coverage. The cost of this coverage is growing rapidly as the population ages and Medicare benefits erode. There has also been a growth of indirect health-related programs such as workers' compensation and short- and long-term disability insurance progams.

In recent years, escalating health care costs have forced employers to find new ways of managing their benefits more efficiently. Today employers are more aggressive in arranging for therapeutically efficient and cost-effective care, for instance. There is increasing stress on benefit redesign, data analysis and cost control, utilization review, alternative provider arrangements, employer coalitions, self insurance, and second opinion programs. By offering cost-effective quality care, companies can maximize the health and productivity of their employees.

OCCUPATIONAL SAFETY AND HEALTH

The first occupational health programs developed independently of the insurance companies as early as the 1900s, and were initiated for a variety of reasons, many unrelated to health. Smoking policies, safety regulations, and recreation programs were implemented for morale and product quality reasons, not for health benefits.

By the 1940s, companies begain focusing on the work environment as a major source of occupational health problems. Agriculture, natural resources, and manufacturing dominated the economy. Attention was paid to occupational hazards associated with these industries, such as chemical carcinogens, asbestos and exposure to coal and cotton dust. Various programs were designed to reduce the incidence of injuries, illnesses and deaths attributable to these causes. The movement received strong federal support in the late 1960s with the passage of the Coal Mine Health and Safety Act of 1969 and the Occupational Safety and Health Act of 1970.

Today the occupational health field is stronger than ever, bringing together the fields of toxicology, industrial hygiene, environmental epidemiology, and occupational medicine. The threat of worksite and toxic chemical exposures still looms high in many workplaces, particularly exposure to new chemicals that are not immediately obvious. Many of these agents are in fact coming from the emerging electronics and biotechnology industries.

PREVENTION AND WELLNESS

The changing nature of illness, from acute infectious diseases to lifestyle-related disorders, and the growing connection between employee health and productivity are primarily responsible for the growth of worksite wellness and prevention. The first of these programs began as early as the 1940s, either focusing on a single illness such as alcoholism, or on a single sector in the workforce, such as a provision for executive physicals. By the 1970s, the idea became popularly known as "worksite wellness," and began expanding in many directions involving the expertise of corporate medical directors, employee assistance counselors, and health education specialists. Specific program examples include health risk assessment, drug and alcohol counseling, smoking cessation, fitness, and stress management.

Worksite wellness is based on the following principles:

- Growing scientific evidence about prevention. Over 50 percent of disease is caused by lifestyle risk factors such as poor diet, smoking, sedentariness, excessive stress, and obesity.
- A focus on general health and disease, not just health that is directly work-related.
- A focus on the individual, rather than the work environment, as a major source of health problems and as the target of intervention.

Today, worksite wellness is less a curiosity and more the norm in many companies. Several national surveys document the growth in the number and variety of programs. Companies report that these programs serve as employee benefits, employee relations tools, productivity enhancers, cost containment strategies, and human resource programs. Unions are increasingly receptive. There is also a growing body of research supporting the cost-effectiveness of wellness and prevention at the workplace.

HUMAN RESOURCE DEVELOPMENT

In a short 25 years the status of the personnel officer has changed from employment manager to top executive with expertise in human capital management. This elevation in status occurred independent of the health function inside companies. Several forces contributed to the change, including:

- The need for increased employer productivity when faced with increasing national and international competition.
- The growth of government regulations covering equal employment opportunity, income maintenance, privacy, industrial relations, compensation, and occupational safety and health.
- An increasing recognition that the key resource in an information/service economy is information, knowledge, and creativity — each embodied in employees.

- The need to conserve an organization's human resources, especially in a competitive labor market where the best and brightest gravitate to companies with the most enlightened human resource programs.
- Expanding knowledge of behavioral and managerial sciences.
- A greater appreciation for training, education, leadership, organizational development and quality of worklife.
- A greater need for human resource planning and cost accounting.
- An increasing sophistication about human resource data systems.
- Changing attitudes and values among employees.

Today human resource management is a total system involving planning, selecting, developing, and evaluating employees. The human resources professional oversees a number of interdependent functions:

- Union and labor relations
- Compensation and benefits
- Wage and salary adminstration
- Performance planning and arbitration
- Training and development
- Management development
- Organizational development
- Personnel and career planning
- Selection and recruitment

A REVOLUTION IN ORGANIZATIONAL HEALTH

The four areas outlined above have contributed significantly to the growth of the organizational health field in several ways. First, employees, dependents, and retirees now have immediate access to a sophisticated health care system, primarily through employer-subsidized health care benefits. Second, an expanding occupational safety and health field has attempted, with varying degrees of success, to minimize toxic exposures in the workplace, many considered primary sources of occupational problems. Third, an increasing number of companies are initiating wellness and prevention activities in the belief that workers leading healthy lifestyles can reduce health care costs. Finally, company human resource strategies are slowly being examined from a health perspective.

Healthy Companies—13

Unfortunately, most policies in this area have focused almost exclusively on performance and productivity, not health.

Despite their accomplishments, the four divisions described above are limited, both individually and collectively, in their approach to health at the workplace because each focuses on only one aspect of the larger problem. In most cases there is minimal interaction across departments, and little appreciation for the connection between corporate culture and employee health.

The healthy corporation, by retaining the strengths of each of these departments while compensating for their limitations, offers an integrated approach for organizations. From this perspective, health and human resource management are viewed as complementary, working in concert toward health and productivity.

Part I

What Is the Healthy Company?

The concept of the "healthy corporation" is a synthesis of fifty years of research on health and human resources in the workplace. The concept links individual health with profitability, as well as with all the potential that lies in connecting these two important goals. It puts dollar figures on people, applying the concept of health and human capital to a company's most valued resources — namely its employees.

As John Naisbitt pointed out in his book *Re-Inventing the Corporation*, "Human capital replaces dollar capital as the strategic resource where people and profits are inexorably linked." From this perspective we can see how knowledge, creativity, and commitment directly relate to employee health and how together they affect performance and the bottom line.

1

Key Considerations of the "Healthy Corporation"

The healthy corporation takes an integrated view of health and the organization.

Four elements in particular are critical:

- The impact of the employee's lifestyle on his or her own health
- The impact of the work environment on the employee's health
- The impact of employee health on the organization's profitability
- The impact of the larger environment — family, peers, leisure — on employee health and organizational profits.

EMPLOYEE'S IMPACT ON HEALTH

The changing nature of most illnesses from acute, infectious disease to chronic, degenerative illnesses suggests that the major causes of premature morbidity and death are diseases that can be prevented through lifestyle changes. One in ten employees suffer from two or more "controllable lifestyle risk factors," each strongly related to increased risk of illness and increased costs. Among employees in a typical organization, for examples:

- 29% smoke cigarettes
- 15-25% are hypertensive

- 20-30% are overweight
- 80% underexercise
- 10-20% have mental health problems/substance abuse
- 30% are prone to low-back injury
- 35-45% burn out on the job

Unhealthy stress is a major risk factor for illness as well. Yet stress is a more ubitquitous concept than the other risk factors and unique for a variety of reasons.

- Stress can be positive or negative. It is important to differentiate between stress that is challenging and stimulating, and stress that is debilitating and a threat to health and well-being.
- Stress can exacerbate all other lifestyle risk factors.
- Stress is associated with a range of physical and mental disorders. Indeed, most medical textbooks attribute anywhere from 50 to 80 percent of all disease to stress-related origins.
- Physical disorders in which unhealthy stress has been implicated include colds, minor infections, bronchial asthma, hypertension, immune disease, peptic ulcer, hyperthyroidism, cardiovascular illness, cancer, and female reproductive dysfunction.
- Impressive evidence also suggests that excessive stress is a risk factor in the precipitation of mental disorders, such as depression, anxiety, schizophrenia, sleep disturbances, alcoholism, and drug abuse.
- Various physical, psychological, and environmental conditions are capable of producing unhealthy stress.
- Stress-related disorders may be acute and transient, or persistent and enduring.
- The outcomes of prolonged excessive stress may be physiological, psychological, behavioral, organizational, and financial.

IMPACT OF WORK ENVIRONMENT ON HEALTH

The environment in which one works is an important causal factor in the development of physical and mental disorders. There are several ways to examine this connection. The National Institute for Occupational Safety and Health (NIOSH) compiled a list of the leading work-related diseases and injuries in the United States. NIOSH used three measurements in compiling this list: how often the diseases or injuries occur, how severe they are, and how amenable the causes are to change for the better. "Unhealthy" stress was implicated in each of the ten categories.

1. **Occupational lung diseases** — asbestosis, byssinosis, silicosis, lung cancer, occupational asthma.
2. **Musculoskeletal injuries** — disorders of the back, trunk, upper extremity, neck, lower extremity; traumatically induced injuries.
3. **Occupational cancers (other than lung)** — leukemia, mesothelioma, cancers of the nose, liver, and bladder.
4. **Amputations, fractures, eye loss, lacerations.**
5. **Cardiovascular diseases** — hypertension, coronary artery disease, acute myocardial infarction.
6. **Disorders of reproduction** — infertility, spontaneous abortion, birth defects.
7. **Neurotoxic disorders** — peripheral neuropathy, toxic encephalitis, psychoses, extreme personality changes.
8. **Noise-induced loss of hearing.**
9. **Dermatologic (skin) conditions** — dermatoses, burns, contusions.
10. **Psychological disorders** — neuroses, personality disorders, alcoholism, drug dependency.

The connection between working conditions and health can also be examined by looking at the relationship between the work environment, health problems and productivity. For example, there is now ten years of government-sponsored research documenting the direct impact of organizational policies and procedures on the stress and health problems of workers. It was found that unhealthy organizational stress can result from:

- Too much or too little responsibility.
- Not being able to utilize personal talents or abilities effectively or to full potential.
- Lack of control or authority over job decisions.
- Crowding or social isolation.
- Poor supervision.
- Tense work relationships.
- Impaired communications and lack of opportunity to voice complaints.
- Confusion about one's job or role in the organization.
- Inadequate rewards and promotions.

- Constant change, dull repetition, or job insecurity.
- Unpleasant environmental conditions such as smoking, noise, air pollution, or commuting difficulties.
- Perceived threat of deadly toxic exposures.

Burnout is a condition caused by chronic organizational stress. Experts believe that as many as 35-45 percent of workers suffer from this condition. Many of the work situations described above have been directly linked to burnout.

IMPACT OF EMPLOYEE HEALTH ON ORGANIZATIONAL PROFITABILITY

Human resource specialists and corporate health professionals are able to measure the impact on the bottom line of stress and health problems like the following:

- Job dissatisfaction
- Decreased motivation
- Poor morale
- Burnout
- Lack of commitment to product quality
- Lateness
- Early departures
- Extended lunches
- Decreased quality and quantity of output
- Increased errors
- Missed deadlines
- Work slowdown
- Poor decision making
- Group conflict
- Tense work relations
- Strikes
- Grievances
- Increased transfer and demotion costs
- Accidents
- Time lost due to medical visits
- Disciplinary proceedings
- Excitability
- EEO complaints

- Tense customer relations
- Fatigue
- Hypersensitivity to criticism
- Mental blocks
- Premature retirement
- Poor interpersonal communication
- Forgetting appointments
- Unscheduled machine downtime due to employee tampering
- Absenteeism
- Turnover
- Reduced productivity
- Excessive health-care costs
- Short — and long-term disability
- Workers' compensation premiums
- Accidents
- Early pension payments

As companies become more sophisticated in health and human resource cost accounting, the link between health and the bottom line will become even clearer.

IMPACT OF LARGER ENVIRONMENT ON EMPLOYEE HEALTH AND ORGANIZATIONAL PROFITS

There is a growing awareness that organizational life is connected to other aspects of people's lives, including family, peer groups, leisure activities, and education. General health and occupational health are becoming blurred. Today, companies see the connection between *stress at work and stress at home.*

Americans are redefining the work-nonwork relationship, trying new ways of balancing work, leisure, family life, and career growth. The exaggeration of one area at the expense of another can create an imbalance in one's life — and act as a health threat, resulting in decreased productivity.

2

Trends Affecting Companies

History shows that successful companies are the ones that respond most effectively to changing social, economic and market forces. Successful companies identify future trends and create products and work climates that incorporate these trends into their corporate goals.

Below is a list of just such trends. All organizations will be affected by these changes. Some will respond better than others, incorporating these trends into their goals and creating a healthier, more productive workforce. These will be the "healthy companies." Others will be less visionary, and in all likelihood, less healthy and less competitive.

RISE IN SERVICE AND INFORMATION ECONOMY

The U.S. shift from an industrial manufacturing economy to an economy based on information services and technology has brought about many changes. In 1962, 43 percent of the workforce was in the service sector. By 1985, these professional, technical, clerical, and service personnel accounted for the largest portion of the workforce. By 1995, this figure will have risen to 57 percent.

The nature of work has obviously changed. The mass production-oriented industrial economy relied on uniformity to produce results. The new service and information economy replaces regimented work processes with flexibility and dynamic work groups. Even in the blue collar sector, mechanization and automation will make work more professional and technical.

In the new corporation, creativity is valued. The structure of work is moving from the manipulation of physical objects to mental activities and customer service. These changes are focusing our attention on the interpersonal and psychological aspects of work, and the impact of information technologies on health.

PUSH TOWARD DECENTRALIZATION AND SELF-MANAGEMENT

Many companies are now rejecting bureaucratic, top-heavy management structures for a more decentralized approach to management. Worksites are decreasing in size and companies are moving toward a system where employees and work groups manage themselves. Computers are taking information out of the hands of managers and placing it in the hands of employees. Employers are recognizing that workers know the most about their jobs, blurring the usual distinctions between worker and supervisor. Networks and new corporate structures such as cross-disciplinary teams and independent business units are replacing traditional hierarchies. Over time this trend is likely to have a positive impact on employee health by offering increasing control over work. However, this trend also suggests less need for supervisors. Middle management positions are decreasing — having fallen over 15 percent since 1979 — and this trend will continue. These numbers are disturbing because the number of men and women between 35 and 45, the prime age range for entering middle management, will increase 42 percent between 1985 and 1995. Blocked career paths, health breakdowns, and lapses in productivity are inevitable.

CHANGING VALUE OF WORK

Employees are changing their work attitudes, moving away from the Puritan work ethic and toward quality of life as an important factor both on and off the job. Personal satisfaction, self-expression, and the right to control one's work are now regarded by many as a basic condition of a well-adjusted life.

Social researchers describe this phenomenon as a societal shift toward "expressive values," characterized as an interest in self-growth, a desire for autonomy and participation, a quest for social support, the rejection of authority, and the placement of self-expression ahead of status. These new values have affected worker attitudes and motivation.

For instance, a 1983 Public Agenda Foundation study identified the top ten qualities people want in a job:

- Interesting work
- Recognition for good work
- Chance to develop skills
- Work with people who treat one with respect
- A chance to think for one's self rather than just carry out instructions
- See the end results of one's work
- Work for efficient managers
- Feel well informed about what is going on
- Opportunity to perform a job that is not too easy

This research shows that employees want more from their workplace in the form of increasing rights *and* responsibilities. They want jobs that provide flexibility, autonomy, security, and recognition, and they want opportunities to use their intelligence and skills for personal and career growth. They want ownership, income, and input into the job and the product.

Unfortunately, the vast majority of our workplaces do not satisfy these values and interests. In fact, many believe that the current declines in productivity and job satisfaction are the direct result of an inadequate response by American companies to these changing values.

It is not surprising that the balance of work and leisure is also changing, with employees asking for new kinds of work options, including a declining length of work week, an increase in part-time work, careers alternating between work and "nonwork" periods, variable work schedules and work-at-home.

CHANGING ROLE OF MANAGERS

The role of managers is changing from that of director and order-giver to that of facilitator and coach. One reason for this change is that American workers are rejecting traditional authoritarian management as abrasive and coercive, and are now more interested in collaborative relations, participative management, and authority exercised with restraint and respect for the employee.

Some employers are seeing the benefits of enlightened management, and in these companies, a new set of skills is required to ensure the success of managers. The new manager must be facilitator, mentor, and leader all in one to cultivate the full potential of subordinates.

Interestingly, the practice of management is also being viewed as either health-promoting or stress-producing, implicating management style and specific qualities of the individual manager as one cause of employee burnout.

CHANGING DEMOGRAPHICS

Shifts from blue collar to white collar, and from younger to older workers, and increases in the number of working women, minorities, and disabled workers, have all diversified the workforce. Many of these groups have special needs to which companies must respond to ensure their health and productivity.

- Americans are aging. In 1980, 20 percent of the population was over 65 years of age. By 2000, this number should reach 23 percent, and by 2020 33 percent of the population will be considered elderly.
- Now nearly 55 percent of women work compared with only 38 percent in 1960, and only 27 percent in 1940. Virtually all women in their 20s and 30s work unless they have small children. Over one half with children under six work. By 1990, it is estimated that women will constitute 50 percent of the workforce and that 80 percent of these women will have children.
- Changes in family structure will also have an impact. Already, in 1985, traditional families, defined as working husband and homebound wife, account for only 10 percent. The future is likely to bring continued growth in two-career families, single-parent families, and males and females in new social and economic roles.
- Almost 15 percent of the working-age population is disabled to some extent. Eleven million people, nearly half of all working-aged disabled, are severely disabled. 44 percent of working-age disabled men are unemployed, and 70 percent of all disabled women remain outside the workforce.

- Blacks, Hispanics, Pacific-Asian Americans, and American Indians — the generally recognized U.S. minorities — are at the highest risk of occupational illness. One recent study reported that black workers have a 37 percent greater risk than whites of suffering an occupational injury or illness and a 20 percent greater chance of dying from job related disorders.

NEW OPPORTUNITIES FOR PREVENTION

The traditional view that health is merely the absence of disease is shifting toward the perception that optimal health can be achieved through environmental safety, organizational changes, and personal lifestyles.

By expanding our view of health, Americans now see disease prevention and health promotion as an essential ingredient in a healthy and productive life. Several trends are responsible for this shift.

- The changing nature of disease from acute infectious illnesses to chronic, lifestyle related disorders.
- The recognition that behavioral and environmental interventions have the greatest potential for improving health.
- The expanding knowledge about stress, mental health, and mind-body interactions.
- The increasing acceptance of self-care and prevention by employees and their families.
- The increased employer understanding about prevention, increased evidence of the cost-effectiveness of prevention programs generally, and worksite programs specifically.
- The recognition that the worksite is a major source of "unhealthy" stress.

GROWING INTEREST IN HUMAN CAPITAL

Traditionally, workplaces have been designed to maximize efficiency and short-term profits, often at the expense of human capital. But today, changing trends and perceptions, in combination with escalating labor and health care costs, have led many employers to view their employees as a form of capital to be nurtured. The growing employer interest in human resource development, wellness, training, and worker participation are examples of this changing focus.

Developments in health and human resource data systems have also helped to advance the field by making available more information about people. Companies can now begin to link streams of "human" information (e.g., occupational risks, health insurance claims, organizational climate, health risk information, performance ratings, absenteeism, turnover), enabling them to study the connection between employee health, work performance, and organizational climate. In the future, analyses like these will distinguish healthy from unhealthy corporations.

INCREASING UNION SUPPORT

Union officials have generally been suspicious of "unhealthy companies," claiming that corporate health and human resource programs often "blame the victim" without paying close enough attention to organizational change. Unions view job stress as related to workplace conditions, rather than to unhealthy workers, and contend that complaints about stress are actually signs of health. Unions are more concerned about the lack of control over work content, unrealistic task demands, lack of understanding by management, and anxiety about job security as primary causes of work stress.

For these reasons, the concept of the healthy corporation may be attractive to unions in the future, primarily because employees and employers in these organizations will share in the responsibility for workplace health problems.

LEGAL INVOLVEMENT IN WORKERS' HEALTH

Increasingly, employees are bringing legal suit against companies for diseases thought to be induced at the worksite. Stress-related illness and progressive occupational disease are receiving the most attention. For instance,

- A Michigan assembly-line worker, unable to keep up with his production line's speed and subjected to frequent barrages of criticism from his supervisor, suffered a psychological breakdown. The court awarded compensation, ruling that the worker's psychosis was caused by the chronic emotional pressures of his job.

- A Boston employee with 22 years' seniority suffered a nervous breakdown when told she would be transferred to another department. The Massachussetts Supreme Judicial Court ruled 4 to 3 that she was entitled to workers' compensation benefits. Her breakdown was a "personal injury arising out of and in the course of . . . employment," the court explained.

What began as a trickle of job-stress claims in the late 1970s has swelled steadily, expanding the liability of a workers' compensation system that already dispenses more than $18 billion a year in benefits. A 1984 13-state study completed by the National Council on Compensation Insurance showed that 11 percent of the workers' compensation claims filed annually for occupational diseases from 1980 through 1982 were for stress.

There are now three types of mental-disability stress cases: physical injury resulting in a mental disorder; mental trauma resulting in physical damage; and mental trauma resulting in mental disorder. Increasingly, state workers' compensation laws are permitting compensation for inquiries resulting from continued stress on the job. In California, for instance, the number of mental-stress inquiries reported to the workers' compensation board more than tripled from 1,282 in 1980 to 4,236 in 1984.

There is a growing acceptance in the medical community of the direct connection between workplace stress and such illnesses as heart disease, hypertension, peptic ulcers, migraines, depression, and suicidal tendencies. Most troubling is that employees of today are increasingly convinced of the link between workplace stress and illness. Younger people know about psychological ills, often are unashamed of them, and are more willing to view their emotional problems as compensable injuries.

3

Principles of Healthy Companies

Several principles distinguish the healthy corporation from other types of organizations. For one thing, healthy companies are divided into seven environments, with considerable overlap among them. These include the physical, psychosocial, emotional, medical, organizational, economic, and community environments. Each of these environments defines health in its own language and measures health by its own yardsticks. The goal, however, is the same across environments: To maximize individual health and organizational profitability.

Healthy companies are flexible and open to changing — changing workers, changing jobs, changing management styles, changing organizational climates, changing policies.

Healthy companies are only as healthy as their parts, namely employees, managers, executives, unions, dependents, and retirees. They enlist the participation, support and expertise of all relevant departments, something that often requires an examination of corporate culture, management, and communication patterns inside a company. The following departments should be represented:

- Top Management
- Medical
- Benefits and compensation
- Employee relations
- Human resource development

- Training and organizational development
- Environmental safety and health
- Line management
- Health education/Employee assistance
- Unions
- Legal

Healthy companies understand the connection between work conditions and health. They realize that policies and company practices can either promote health and productivity, or produce stress, burnout, and excessive healthcare costs. They fully appreciate the direct link between health and human resource management, as well as the inter-connection among health, morale, and productivity.

Healthy companies exhibit the proper degree of stress that stimulates employee performance and a quality worklife. Ultimately these are tied to the following:

- Work conditions
- Opportunities for participation and decision-making
- Work relationships
- Opportunities for career growth
- Clear work roles
- Well-managed change

Healthy companies believe that people who are well managed are healthier, and that healthier people produce better results. Explicitly, they support the activities of the medical department through a positive corporate environment.

Healthy companies avoid single-purpose and short-term solutions, and take a long-term perspective on their employees. Their approach is proactive, not reactive.

Healthy companies understand that what is healthy for some may be unhealthy for others. They tailor their approach to the culture of the workforce population, recognizing the importance of matching individual needs with specific health and human resources programs. For example, Type A, achievement-oriented employees are potentially at risk for health problems when they are managed by supervisors who provide inadequate freedom to make decisions and impose excessive guidance and structure.

Healthy companies are run on top-down and bottom-up approaches. Leadership, commitment, and investment from top management are critical, but bottom-up approaches are necessary to create feelings of ownership and family. Employees need to feel control over their work lives.

Healthy companies take advantage of implementing broad environmental and organizational changes. Examples range from nutritious food in the company cafeteria, positive policies regarding mistakes and risk taking, and flexible work scheduling. Healthy companies support values like risk taking, creativity, openness, fairness, team spirit, trust, mutual respect, commitment to excellence, safety, and rights tied to responsibility.

Finally, healthy companies respect the personal and especially the family needs of workers. Their company policies respond to the changing societal values and the changing nature of the American family.

Part II

Diagnosing Corporate Culture

There are seven factors inside organizations not commonly thought of as related to health that place workers at potential risk for health breakdowns:

- Stressful work conditions
- Lack of control/participation
- Tense work relationships
- Lack of career progress
- Unclear work roles
- Poorly managed change
- Family and leisure conflicts

Every work group, department, and division inside a company can be evaluated according to these seven criteria, either alone or in combination with other factors. Some of these conditions are more unhealthy than others, depending on an employee's overall health and whether there are positive counteracting forces inside the company. Generally these factors have a negative long-term effect on employee health and productivity. The more factors present, the greater the risk.

There are two basic corporate strategies that can be used to improve employee health and productivity. One is to increase a worker's resistance to sickness through offering wellness and prevention opportunities, such as stress management, smoking cessation, hypertension control, nutrition education, and weight control programs. The other strategy is to create a work climate that promotes health and productivity through human resource policies and programs. A combination of the two will ultimately produce the most healthy corporate culture, but here we will focus solely on the second of these two strategies.

The link between organizational climate and health has received the least amount of attention, despite well-documented evidence that a healthy work climate is critical to the "healthy corporation." By creating an atmosphere that promotes health and productivity, companies can support their other "health-related activities," such as health benefits and wellness programs, through health-promoting personnel programs and policies. Without this supporting climate, organizations potentially sabotage their investments in human capital by creating unhealthy workplaces that ultimately cause unnecessary health breakdowns among employees.

4

Stressful Work Conditions

Traditionally, concern about work-related dangers has been limited to blue collar workers in manufacturing settings. The threat of occupational injuries is still high in these settings and continues to require careful monitoring. But, the focus on blue collar work has diverted our attention away from the stressful nature of work conditions generally, and the growing dangers associated with white collar jobs in particular.

For example, the nature of work often goes unnoticed as a source of health risk. For instance, when employees are asked to perform too much work without adequate resources, little attention is paid to the health effects. Examples of such work overload include excessively paced machines, speed-ups, and unreasonable physical demands like unrealistic deadlines and time pressures. The secretary bombarded with excessive demands and the factory employee driven by uncontrollable automation both work under these conditions. Instructions by intrusive supervisors, demands by co-workers, understaffing, and excessive control of work by company rules can exacerbate the problem.

At the other end of the continuum, many jobs underutilize human knowledge, skills, and initiative. Monotonous work with little responsibility, narrow content, little variation, and low demands on creativity exemplify this type of work. Workers performing these tasks view themselves as powerless to cope with the fractionation of their work and the impersonal nature of their organizations. The result is alienation, stress, and a lack of commitment. Jobs like these exist throughout the technology, service, and manufacturing sectors.

Crowded working conditions and lack of privacy can also have deleterious effects on employee health. Inadequate physical and psychological space leads to feelings of confinement, tense interpersonal relations, and stress for all around. Examples of workers in this category include coal miners, employees who must wear confining body apparatus, and clerical staff working in open, densely populated offices. Isolating jobs, such as that of a security guard, can also lead to feelings of alienation, loneliness, and stress.

Perhaps the greatest occupational hazard of all is the modern white-collar office building. Some commonly cited office risk factors include inappropriate lighting, poor air quality, extreme temperature variations, noise pollution, and poorly designed equipment.

Inappropriate lighting design can include excess lighting, inefficient lighting, and glare. Poor air quality can be caused by indoor air pollutants such as micro-organisms, cigarette smoke, dust, and poor ventilation. Chemical emissions from machines include ozone from photocopiers, methyl and alcohol from mimeographs, ammonia from blueprint machines, and formaldehyde from carbonless copy paper. Unhealthy noise can originate with office machines, ventilation systems, and conversation. The cumulative effects of these, and the psychological stress associated with them, is poorly understood.

RESEARCH FINDINGS

Various research links stressful work conditions to health and productivity problems. A number of important areas are reviewed below.

Negative Physical Environment

Every year, one out of every nine workers in private industry will suffer an occupational injury — over five million injuries. Latest Department of Health & Human Services figures show nearly 14,000 workers die in job accidents each year, and more than 2.5 million workers are disabled by injuries, over 100,000 of them permanently.

Approximately 21 million American workers are exposed to substances regulated by the Occupational Safety and Health Administration. The National Cancer Institute and the National Institute of Environmental Health Services reports that 20 percent of all future cancers will be related to workplace exposures. Other studies have estimated that as many as 14 million workers are exposed daily to toxic materials.

Work Overload/Too Much Work With Inadequate Resources

In a recent NIOSH study listing the most stressful occupations by their relationship to disease, the one similarity between almost all of the jobs was the fast pace of work with little chance of relief.

Research has shown that work overload is associated with increased hypertension, heart attacks, job dissatisfaction, anxiety, depression, drinking, absenteeism, decreased self esteem, and numerous family difficulties. The greatest physical and mental health difficulties occur when work overload and skill underutilization are combined.

A study of workers under the age of 45 in light industry showed that those who worked more than 48 hours a week had twice the risk of death due to heart disease compared to those working a 40-hour week. Other studies have correlated long working hours with such indicators of stress as absenteeism, drinking, low motivation, and low self-esteem.

A study of office workers whose jobs involved frequent overtime work found that increased epinephrine levels (a physiological sign of increased stress) were present both during and after working hours. Another classic study showed marked increases in the blood cholesterol levels of tax accountants as the April 15 filing deadline approached. After the deadline, their cholesterol levels gradually returned to normal.

Various types of research link excessive job demands to morbidity and mortality. For example, in a ten-year study workers with high job demands at two points in time (two years apart) were three times as likely to die in the next decade than workers with either high demands at only one point or low demands at the same points in time.

Repetitious/Monotonous Work

There is an extensive literature showing that repetition, monotony, and a lack of variation is related to poor health, from hypertension and cardiovascular risk to excessive drinking and depression.

According to a study of 2,000 people at the University of Michigan's Institute for Occupational Safety, those who reported being bored at work felt that their abilities were not being used and that their job did not promise as much complexity and variety as they wanted. These conditions frustrated their desire to perform well, causing unnecessary stress that was harmful to their productivity and their health.

Shiftwork

Research in the last 20 years has clearly established the existence of rhythms that regulate the fluctuation of many of the body's systems such as hormone levels, temperature, and blood pressure within a 24 hour period. The peak of the body's activity is in the middle of the day and lowest activity is at night. The problem for shift workers is that these internal body rhythms do not match the demands of their workday.

Studies show that shiftwork upsets the body's 24-hour rhythms, leading to fatigue, increased accidents, less-than-optimum job performance, worker dissatisfaction, and increased health problems. Other studies have indicated higher frequencies of sleep, mood, and digestive disturbances among shift workers than among constant-day workers. Shift workers have also been found to be more susceptible to the effects of physical agents like noise, vibration, radiation, and chemical agents like fumes, gases, and dusts.

Rotating shift workers have a higher incidence of ulcers than workers in steady day or night shifts. Research suggests that proper chrono hygiene (planned rescheduling of meals and activities) and appropriate shift schedules minimize physiological and sociological problems. Long-term benefits of these programs include higher morale, fewer accidents, improved health, and higher productivity.

Noise

Studies repeatedly demonstrate that noise pollution is a major health risk and an important deterrent to productivity. More than 20 million workers are exposed to "hazardous" noise every year. It has been estimated that almost three quarters of the workers who spend 20 years on their jobs under current allowable noise levels will experience hearing loss, and studies in noisy industries have shown that cases of ulcers were as much as five times as numerous as normally would be expected.

Ventilation

The incidence of health problems related to office air has risen dramatically with the widespread adoption of tightly sealed energy-efficient office buildings. Dangerous build-ups of toxic substances and bacteria have been linked to numerous symptoms and illnesses.

Office machinery and equipment give off hazardous fumes that are often circulated in small windowless rooms. Many office workers are plagued by headaches, fatigue, and other problems that are signals of improper ventilation. The General Accounting Office reports that higher concentrations of air pollutants have been found in indoor as compared to outdoor environments. More than 770,000 American workers are exposed to ionizing radiation on their jobs via x-ray machines, radioactive material, laser beams, and electronic equipment. A NIOSH study showed that a simple duplicating machine can give off methyl alcohol vapors in concentrations nearly four times the recommended exposure limits. This can cause nausea, dizziness, blurred vision, and skin problems.

Steel and glassworkers who work at high temperatures for prolonged periods of time have enlarged hearts and higher rates of arteriosclerosis than other working populations. Lost time due to sickness was increased by 63 percent for miners working at 80 degrees Farenheit compared to a similar group working at 70 degrees.

Video Display Terminals (VDTs)

Prolonged use of video display terminals (VDTs) has been shown to be directly linked to musculoskeletal, cardiovascular, and visual problems. Musculoskeletal disorders have been one of the major categories of self-reported complaints by VDT workers, a high percentage of whom report pains, stiffness, cramps, and numbness in the back, neck, shoulders, arms, and hands. There is also a suggested association between the length of time at the VDT and the level of reported musculoskeletal symptoms.

A study by scientists at the National Institute of Occupational Safety and Health of clerical workers reported that 25 percent of the operators of keyboard machines who were studied suffered from occupational cervicobrachial syndrome, which produces cramps. Another 50 percent of the keyboard operators complained of muscular distress. A Finnish study found that if data-entry workers were trained to recognize these ergonomic problems and to prevent them, the level of neck, shoulder, and elbow problems was significantly reduced over a six-month period.

In a cross-sectional study of clerical workers in the communications industry, those who worked at the VDT were about twice as likely to develop angina pectoris. This was the first study to demonstrate a relationship between automated office work and a valid precursor of cardiovascular disease. Most studies show that support staff who work at a VDT report more psychosomatic symptoms than either other support staff who do not work at VDTs and professionals who do.

Fifteen years of research has shown that VDT workers report a high prevalence of visual strain, ranging in studies between 47 and 91 percent of all operators. VDT work is associated with an increase in visual problems across most occupations, but especially in those with heavy visual demands. There is evidence that work at a VDT leads to more frequent changes in eye glasses, for example. Some have attributed this to the aging of the workers and to a greater tendency for VDT workers, as compared to others, to identify minor visual problems.

Stressful Occupations

A study by scientists at the National Institute of Occupational Safety and Health analyzed Tennessee hospital and death records to determine which jobs rated high in stress-related illnesses, including heart attacks, ulcers, arthritis, and mental disorders. Of 130 jobs studied, these were the twelve highest:

12 Jobs with Most Stress

1. Laborer
2. Secretary
3. Inspector
4. Clinical lab technician
5. Office manager
6. Foreman
7. Manager/administrator
8. Waitress/waiter
9. Machine operator
10. Farm owner
11. Miner
12. Painter

Other High-Stress Jobs

Bank teller	Nurses' aide
Clergyman	Plumber
Computer programmer	Policeman
Dental assistant	Practical nurse
Electrician	Public-relations person
Fireman	Railroad switchman
Guard/watchman	Registered nurse
Hairdresser	Sales manager
Health aide	Sales representative

Health technician	Social worker
Machinist	Structural-metal worker
Meat-cutter	Teacher's aide
Mechanic	Telephone operator
Musician	Warehouse worker

Control Data Corporation (CDC), Minneapolis, Minnesota, reports that in its annual in-house employee health survey, the problem "stress/anxiety/tension" always is at the top of the list, checked by nearly one-third of their employees. CDC has used the same survey with more than thirty other companies and has had the same responses — stress always tops the list of health problems. At New York Telephone, a stress-symptom check list found that 24 percent of participating employees had stress-related symptoms of sufficient severity to warrant intervention, and ten percent of the group needed psychiatric help.

Studies of employee burnout indicate that as many as 45 percent of workers experience the condition at any one time. Burnout is characterized by insomnia, physical complaints, a depressed emotional state, and increased reliance on alcohol and drugs. The condition afflicts all occupations.

CORPORATE APPROACHES

The following is a sampling of some corporate programs designed to protect workers against the effects of unhealthy work conditions. They include:

- Job redesign
- Redesign of physical setting
- Improved safety and hygiene programs
- Job complexity/enlargement/rotation opportunities
- Stress management considerations in defining work tasks

A. Job Redesign

Northwestern Mutual Life Insurance Company

In 1980, Northwestern Mutual Life conducted a study of reporting relationships and work flow in its underwriting and policyowner services departments. It concluded that these operations were too highly specialized and did not maximize the company's large investment in technology. Some analysts were handling only small parts of the underwriting or service functions, without sufficient understanding of the overall process or the role of each function in that process. As a result of the study and with full support from its top management, the company instituted major changes in these departments. Basically, Northwestern changed from a highly functional operation to a "one-stop service," provided through analysts who could complete all or most of the activities related to a particular policy with a high degree of autonomy and with full accountability for the final result.

- Task forces were created to look at each job, each step in the flow of work, and the underlying data processing systems.
- Recognizing that it is critical to involve people when making changes, the company actively sought input from personnel who performed the day-to-day work. Each task force had about six members, ranging from department heads to clerical analysts. As a result of these discussions, accountability was driven downward. Operational functions were regionalized (East, South, Central, West), and each region was given final and complete responsibility for underwriting decisions, issuing policies, and serving the service needs of existing policyowners. Within each region "core jobs" were identified for each function. Before the reorganization, one of these departments had sixty different job descriptions. After reorganization, these were boiled down to six generic jobs. As analysts learned new functions and developed new skills, their job responsibilities were broadened. The company stepped up its training, spending more than 35,000 training hours in 1982 alone.
- To relieve potential tension and stress, Northwestern made a written commitment to its staff, making it clear that no one would lose his or her job because of the reorganization.
- Union leadership was invited to participate in the early discussions, and union observers sat in on training sessions.
- Several important results emerged from the reorganization. Work flow was streamlined, complaints were reduced, and the company reduced the time for processing new applications for insurance. Productivity increased. Morale and job satisfaction improved as 25 percent of those involved in the reorganization

received promotions because of their broadened skills and responsibilities. The company did not have a single union grievance.

B. Redesign of Physical Setting

Herman Miller Inc.

Herman Miller Inc. promotes a concept called "the indeterminate building," an idea that provides opportunity for growth, future options, changes, and a long-standing commitment to participative management and community service. It implies a responsiveness to changing human needs, technology, and individual creativity.

Herman Miller's goal is to make a contribution to the landscape. At each of its facilities, the accent is on green space over constructed space, roughly along these lines:

- 25 percent building
- 25 percent roads/parking
- 50 percent green space

The company also makes a policy of using local, regional, and national sculpture on sites. It tries to make its offices part of the local community. Sites are left open to the community (without fencing) and there is no reserved parking space. Indoor walking space is provided for inclement weather, which is not inconsistent with the goal of encouraging fortuitous encounters and open community. Cafeterias are open to everyone regardless of where they work, and break areas are provided near work spaces in each facility.

The idea is that work space should serve human activity, and there is special concern about lighting levels and ventilation. Building standards are higher than the codes regarding building requirements. Manufacturing plant areas are treated with the same aesthetic concern as are office areas.

Many of Herman Miller's buildings have multiple uses. Each facility must be able to change with grace, be flexible, and nonmonumental. The buildings reflect human scale, using light-weight materials. The company's hope is to create an environment that will be welcoming. Building sites have no fences; their entrances have a sense of arrival.

The quality of the company's work spaces reflects its reputation as a maker of well-designed office environments. Every employee is able to see natural light, for example. The company even burns its own waste to create energy. Herman Miller's facilities are involved with the neighborhood communities. In addition to establishing standards of quality for the buildings in its communities, the company encourages employee participation in civic activities — even if it's only on the level of supporting street improvements.

C. Improved Safety and Hygiene Programs

DuPont

DuPont has one of the most extensive worksite safety programs of any U.S. company. It is a firm policy backed up by extensive company resources.

The overall program was founded on "ten principles of safety."

- All injuries and occupational illnesses can be prevented.
- Management is directly responsible for preventing injuries and illnesses.
- Safety is a condition of employment.
- Training is an essential element for safe workplaces.
- Management must audit safety performance in the workplace.
- All deficiencies must be corrected promptly, either through modifying facilities, changing procedures, bettering employee training, or disciplining constructively.
- It is essential to investigate all unsafe practices and incidents with injury potential.
- Safety off the job is just as important as safety on the job.
- It is good business to prevent illness and injury.
- People are the most critical element in the success of a safety and health program.

DuPont's position on safety is backed up by a written policy stating that the company will not make, handle, use, sell, transport, or dispose of a product unless it can do so safely and in an environmentally sound manner.

At DuPont the chairman of the board is the chief safety officer. He and other senior executives set safety standards and annual safety objectives for the entire company. At worksites worldwide, the individual DuPont manager is personally responsible for the health of each of his subordinates. For example, it is recommended that managers:

- Establish a safety committee and participate in all safety meetings.
- Put safety at the top of the staff meeting agenda.
- Review serious incidents that occur within their offices, as well as incidents that occur in other parts of the company.
- Look for unsafe conditions and take swift corrective action.
- Make safety an integral part of employees' yearly performance reviews.
- Train employees properly.
- Take prompt disciplinary action to correct deficiencies.
- Invest capital resources in protecting people.
- Pay overtime if necessary to correct a safety problem.

Supporting each of these activities are four components of DuPont's occupational health program:

- **Toxicology** — Conducts long- and short-term studies on chemical substances to determine their toxic properties, ranging from skin irritation to carcinogenicity.
- **Industrial hygiene** — Samples and measures the potential risk in the work environment. Noise, for example, or radiation, or contaminants in air and water.
- **Occupational medicine** — Consists of routine and specialized health surveillance and medical care.
- **Epidemiology** — Maintains computerized data files for health surveillance, including mortality of employees and pensioners, employees' disabilities from illness or injury, and a cancer registry to study cancer incidence and mortality.

D. Job Complexity/Enlargement/Rotation Opportunities

Fisher Price

In order to reduce boredom and increase employees' full involvement in their jobs, Fisher Price's production line workers are expected to be able to work on all the various machines in the plant. In fact, workers generally change machines every few hours and work on different portions of a particular toy.

Fisher Price also recognizes the importance of providing an understanding of various engineering disciplines within the company. Consequently, newly recruited engineers rotate over an 18 month period through plastics, product development, and manufacturing engineering.

E. Stress Management Considerations in Defining Work Tasks

IBM

IBM has implemented several programs to help reduce the stressfulness of certain work conditions.

For one, the company applies ergonomic principles at several of its major locations, emphasizing the interrelationships between people and their machines. These principles have two basic objectives: fitting the person to his job and fitting the job to the person. For example, a video training tape and work booklet were prepared for managers at several sites outlining the importance of ergonomic principles. Examples of interventions have included the redesign of factory carts to prevent back strains and sprains; the redesign of rubber hand tools to prevent wrist cramps; and the improved design of VDT's to reduce their glare.

Secondly, IBM educates its managers about the use of visual display terminals. Special attention is given to implementation planning, job design, employee/manager communications, and facility and workplace design.

Rolm Corporation

Rolm has made a special effort to automate the most repetitious, mundane jobs at its manufacturing division. One example includes the use of robotics and carousels to carry parts to various work stations.

Argonne National Labs

At Argonne National Laboratories, the health and performance effects of shiftwork have been studied extensively. Management has used this research to implement a series of programs to improve shift-rotation schedules that minimize the physiological and sociological problems associated with shiftwork.

Experts at Argonne believe that rotations and delays can promote health and adaptation or produce health problems and deteriorating performance. Properly applied "chrono hygiene" can help workers

adjust to these new shifts. Chrono hygiene is th*
of meals and activities, directly manipulating ligh
meal times, and the daily rhythm of rest and activity.
rotation schedules slowly change the body's 24-hour rh
ees never switch more often than by one shift per week. 1
benefits to both employers and employees include higher mo
accidents, improved health, and higher productivity.

5

Lack of Control/Participation

Workers need to feel control over their destinies at home, at work, and in their personal lives. Without this control, some people become alienated or angry, and lose their motivation. Others in the workplace acknowledge their lack of control, but develop a variety of physical and emotional symptoms. In both cases employees feel stressed and disenchanted with their work, placing them at risk for a variety of health problems.

Areas of control important to most people include control over work pace and work methods, process decisions, contact with other people, scheduling, and influence over the planning and design of work. Workers also like to control their potential for failures, disapproval, and future stressors. Unpredictability can be the greatest stress of all, and that can include inconsistent company policies and unpredictable managers.

In recent years, the growth in office automation has expanded the list of jobs that provide little control over work. For instance, when control over when to do a task is determined by a computer system, tasks are said to be machine-paced. When jobs are machine-paced, an office begins to mirror the factory assembly line. Machine pacing can both increase workload and decrease control.

RESEARCH FINDINGS

Numerous studies show that lack of control and limited participation in decision making place workers at risk for a variety of physical and psychological disorders, including increases in somatic symptoms, alcoholism, cardiovascular disease, anxiety, and depression. They are also linked to productivity problems, such as increases in absenteeism and turnover, and decreases in job satisfaction, use of skills, commitment, and creativity.

Laboratory and field studies also show that individuals who can predict, understand, or control events in their organizations experience less organizational stress and are less adversely affected by that stress. Researchers studying workplace stressors found that among a national representative sample of over 1,400 workers, the most significant and consistent predictor of stress was the degree of opportunity to participate in decision making on the job. As opportunities for participation in workplace decisions increased, so did productivity and performance levels. Another survey of 2,300 *Psychology Today* readers, for example, found that respondents overwhelmingly asked for more control over the decisions that affect their jobs.

Cross-sectional, retrospective, and prospective studies all indicate that lack of control over one's work process constitutes an additional risk factor for cardiovascular diseases. In a six-year prospective analysis, men with jobs characterized by a heavy workload and limited job control were found to have 1.4 times the normal risk of cardiovascular disease. In a case-control study of myocardial infarction and occupational exposures, it was found that hectic work and low control over work tempo and skill variety were associated with myocardial infarction in men under 55. In a study of Swedish workers who had changed jobs, those whose new job offered greater control had fewer coronary symptoms than workers whose new job had less control.

A Swedish insurance company found that when the computer system went down, workers responded with increased arousal, higher blood pressure, fatigue, and feelings of being rushed. Further, if the software did not provide the needed information, there was decreased control over the work, producing anxiety and job dissatisfaction.

In an American study, women who described their jobs as heavy in workload with limited job control had a three-fold greater risk of developing coronary heart disease (CHD) as women reporting a heavy workload but having control over their work. (Men did not exhibit the same relationship.) At greatest risk were clerical women, who had a 420 percent greater chance of developing CHD. These associations persisted after controlling for the traditional risk factors for CHD in women.

A recent National Heart, Lung and Blood Institute study showed a 100 percent increase in heart attacks among secretaries, typists, clerks, and bookkeepers when compared to housewives. Working women in general did not appear to be at greater risk than housewives, but those in office occupations were, because they had been placed in situations where they were not able to express anger or emotions, and so literally took their frustration to heart.

A survey of 40,000 working women found that "unhealthy work conditions" were responsible for a wide variety of stress-related disorders, including eye strain, fatigue, insomnia, disgestive problems, anxiety, and depression. Stress illnesses occurred most often in those under the greatest pressure but having the least influence over their work. The two worst working conditions were: (1) a lot of pressure or responsibility without enough authority to make decisions, and (2) no ability to affect how work is done.

Personality research indicates that there are certain types of "stress-resistant" employees who pride themselves on taking control over their work. One study identified these employees by comparing two groups of high stress executives. Both groups had similar jobs in the same company, but one group had the most illnesses and health claims, and one had the least. The healthier group was characterized as stress-resistant. It was found that these stress-resistant executives differed from their less healthy co-workers in three qualities:

- Openness to challenge
- Involvement in work
- Sense of personal control over work.

CORPORATE APPROACHES

Following is a sampling of some corporate programs designed to protect workers against stress and health problems associated with lack of control in the workplace. The goals of these programs are:

1. To move authority from higher to lower levels;
2. To increase the range of skills and abilities of each worker; and
3. To increase shared decision making and rewards.

The programs include:

- Upward communication programs
- Participative/self-management opportunities
- Control over workpace, process decisions and scheduling
- Opportunities for intrapreneurship
- Organization-wide reward/compensation programs

A. Upward Communication Programs

Dana Corporation

Believing that people are its most important asset, Dana is dedicated to encouraging upward communication and minimizing any feelings of powerlessness among employees inside their organization. Principles such as "helping people grow, encouraging entrepreneurship, pushing responsibility down, involving everyone, communicating fully, and breaking down organizational barriers" are examples of the company's commitment.

Dana's policy is based on a two-way model of communication. It is the responsibility of managers and employees to inform each other about activities at Dana. Several programs exemplify these principles:

"Ask Me" is a program that gives employees direct access to top management. Prestamped notepads addressed to the chairman are available in all locations. Employees are asked to communicate directly about any issue with the chairman, and they do: the chairman receives 15 letters per week and responds to each one.

The chairman and the president of Dana's North American Operations also travel thirty days each year to worksites to talk with Dana people about the company's status, and conversely, to receive feedback and answer questions of employees.

Erie Insurance Group

Erie Insurance Group truly believes that an open air of communication can help promote a healthful employee atmosphere. Since its founding in 1925, Erie Insurance has been committed to a philosophy of service and accessibility to both customers and employees. In fact, that philosophy is a cornerstone of Erie's corporate culture. Both of these policies were initiated by Erie Insurance's founder, H.O. Hirt, and have been continued over the years by his successor, F.W. Hirt. All employees, including the chairman, answer their own phones, and policyholders can call any of Erie's executives, including the chairman, collect at any time. The door knocker on the inside of the chairman's door symbolizes Erie's open door policy. His door is always open to meet with agents and employees. This spirit of open communication is enhanced by a number of formal programs. These programs encourage employees to deal directly with any problems they may experience. Supervisors are trained to foster face-to-face communications through such programs as "I Am Concerned" that lists, step by step, the actions that employees must take to resolve their concerns.

Other programs include "The Pipeline" in which employees can raise concerns and propose solutions or improvements. Employees can also make recommendations through a biannual organizational communication audit of the total workforce. Results of this audit are compiled and distributed to every employee. Group meetings are held at various levels to discuss many of the topics raised during the audit.

H.B. Fuller

To promote access to the president and to underscore the importance of employee opinions, especially those of new employees and those of employees from newly acquired companies, Fuller uses a "President's Hotline." Twice a year employees can call direct to the president and discuss issues of concern.

B. Participative/Self-Management Opportunities

W.L. Gore & Associates, Inc.

Emphasizing personal responsibility and personal management, W.L. Gore & Associates, Inc. has devised a unique system of unmanagement whereby "Associates" (personnel are not "employees") are given freedom and opportunity to develop on the job. At Gore, Associates are encouraged to grow in knowledge, skill, and scope of responsibility, and are asked to make voluntary commitments to the organization. In exchange for these commitments, "sponsors" (not "bosses") expose Associates to a full range of opportunities.

There are no formal titles, hierarchies, nor conventional structures at

Gore, nor any assigned authority. Training and supervison are carried out through an informal mentoring process called the Sponsorship Program. Each Associate participates with three different types of sponsors:

- **Starting sponsor** — This sponsor is much like a Big Brother/Sister. His primary responsibility is to indoctrinate new employees, and help them grow into independent, responsible Associates. After one year, Associates are given the opportunity to find new sponsors.
- **Advocate sponsor** — This sponsor plays the role of advocate in all discussions inside the organization. An Associate can have many advocates.
- **Compensation sponsor** — Along with other key personnel, this sponsor determines an Associate's contribution to the success of the enterprise, and decides on salary, compensation, and personnel requests.

Gore Associates learn about the principles of self-management and commitment through the sponsorship process, as well as through more formal ongoing discussion groups.

Ford

At Ford's Edison plant, management and labor, hourly and salaried employees, work together to ensure that the plant is operating to its potential. The process began in 1981, when management and the United Auto Workers agreed to investigate operating problems. This new style of participation represents a real change in attitude toward employees.

At the time, plant management and the union talked to plant personnel to identify problems. An employee involvement program was established, combining a plant-wide open-door policy with problem-solving teams and employee meetings. Teams of hourly and salaried employees received sixteen hours of training in areas including problem-solving techniques, effective listening, and statistical process control. The teams met for one hour every two weeks to address issues affecting product quality, employee satisfaction, working conditions, and the manufacturing process.

Employees now have an opportunity to participate in periodic mass meetings held throughout the plant. Employees can participate to the extent of conducting visitor tours through the plant (for which management frees them for up to two to three hours).

Donnelly Corporation

Donnelly's approach to participative management grew out of its Scanlon Plan. The normal corporate structure and leadership roles are modified to include and encourage a combination of participative management (including participative vs. self-managed teams and problem-solving committees) with profit sharing.

In keeping with its overriding philosophy of individual responsibility, Donnelly employees, operating in teams of ten or more, manage many of their own work activities, which include:

- Setting their own team and individual work goals (consistent with corporate goals)
- Keeping track of their own progress

Policy, equity, and compensation issues are dealt with by employee-elected committees, which meet monthly. Committee members return to work teams to discuss issues and seek recommendations. Decisions of this committee group are final (except for annual salary packages, which go to the board of directors for approval), and are made only by unanimous agreement.

C. Control over Workpace, Process Decisions, and Scheduling

Honeywell

In 1974, Honeywell began a unique participative management program with the goal of improving organizational productivity and the quality of work life. The overall objective was to help employees become more self-determining at work, improve quality, and reduce the tension associated with authoritarian management.

The program is based on the assumption that people want to perform well, and what they need most are opportunities. It asks employees two basic questions:

- What is keeping you from being more productive?
- How can we make this a better place to work?

Today, there are well over 2,000 "Quality Management" systems at Honeywell, 60 percent in factory settings. Groups may meet weekly or once a month. In their discussions they may focus on a wide variety of job-related topics, such as work flow, scheduling, quality improvement, new products, and organizational climate issues. Honeywell reports that its employees are more satisfied, less stressed, and more productive. Absenteeism and accidents are down.

Rolm Corporation

A central philosophy at all Rolm manuacturing facilities is that workers should have maximum control over workpace, work process, and quality control. Rolm aims to accomplish this through the following:

- Training employees in a variety of tasks
- Expanding workers' responsibilities
- Educating workers about the entire work process
- Giving employees control over that process

Rolm employees set up their own tracking and quality control systems, and present the results of this system to fellow employees on a regular basis. All performance is monitored closely and rewarded.

Ford

To ensure product quality at Ford's Edison plant, workers have immediate control over the production process. At any point, workers can halt the entire production line by pushing a button on the line. The production line will be stopped, the problem immediately corrected, and the line restarted — often with only a ten- or twelve-second delay. The use of this system has had some significant benefits:

- The number of defects per car was reduced from 17.1 to 0.8 per car
- The number of cars requiring reworking was reduced 97 percent
- The backlog of union grievances plummeted
- Employee attitudes improved tremendously and employees even began solving problems at home
- The Edison plant consistently ranks first or second in quality of all Ford's production facilities.

Digital Equipment Corporation

Digital operates on two basic assumptions about its employees:

- Workers often know more about their jobs than their managers.
- The individual is responsible for his own career.

According to a Digital manager, "One of the most dehumanizing assumptions ever made is that workers work and managers think. When we give shop floor workers control over their work, they are enormously thoughtful."

Digital workers often create and manage their own jobs. They are encouraged to propose projects and are responsible for their own success. Employees take responsibility for locating their next jobs and determining how and when to move on. Communication at Digital is on a first-name basis and decision-making is frequently done by consensus.

D. Opportunities for Intrapreneurship

Eastman Kodak Company

Started in 1898, Kodak's suggestion program is the oldest continuous program of its kind in the U.S. It is an integral part of the company's business system and is managed by a staff of four full-time personnel.

The suggestion process is simple. Kodak employees are given opportunities to propose new products and solutions to problems by submitting a suggestion of any kind to the Suggestion Office. Subject-matter experts inside the company evaluate the idea and decide its potential applicability. Each suggestion gets a response; there is a 33 percent adoption rate. Cash awards are given to winners, with a maximum award of $50,000.

Employees receive 15 percent of the savings resulting from the suggestion during the first two years. In 1984, Kodak adopted 5,000 safety suggestions alone, paid 21,400 people cash awards, and saved over $12 million. Four employees received the maximum award of $50,000.

3M Company

3M's long-standing commitment to innovation and in-house entrepreneurship is exemplified by the company's philosophy on nurturing creativity, "Thou shalt not kill a new product idea, just deflect it." To stimulate innovations, 3M offers a variety of programs, each designed to give employees opportunities to grow, and create on the job. Below is a list of several:

- **Stimulate boundary crossing.** 3M minimizes the organizational barriers that can impede innovation by fostering communication among its technical, marketing, manufacturing, and human resource divisions. For example, in Austin, Texas, research and marketing people are placed in close physical proximity to encourage collaborative activities.
- **Empower employees.** 3M creates opportunities for employees to innovate entrepreneurally. "Genesis" is a program for scientists and technical personnel in which they have the opportunity to pursue innovative areas of research and are given funds to operate independently. "Venture Career Path" is a new program for in-house entrepreneurs, providing them with staff and sufficient funding to take an embryonic idea all the way to market. "Optimize Operations" is a quality of worklife/quality circle program located in many 3M manufacturing plants.
- **Rewards and recognition.** 3M strives to find new ways of rewarding and recognizing talent inside the corporation. It maintains a promotion-from-within policy and offers dual career paths for scientists in research labs. 3M continues to recognize and financially reward outstanding contributions in the technical area.
- **Smallness and flexibility.** 3M calls itself a "biological" organization. When a new product sells well enough, a new division is born. Median plant size is 114 people, and only five of the 91 U.S. plants have more than 1,000 people.

E. Organization-wide Reward/Compensation Programs

Several types of financial reward programs can be initiated to give employees a sense of control over company profits. Examples include profit sharing, equity and bonus distributions, stock options, Scanlon plans, and cooperative ownership.

Federal Express

Federal Express offers three compensation programs that encourage employees to relate their individual performance to the profits of the company.

- **Current profit sharing plan** — Based on the financial health of the company, every six months a percentage of profits is distributed to employees in cash. This percentage has ranged from 5 percent of salary in December, 1983 (average $825/employee) to 2-3 percent in 1985.
- **Deferred profit sharing plan** — Through the deferred profit sharing plan, the company makes annual contributions, in cash or stock, to the individual accounts of employees.
- **Employee stock ownership plan** — Through an employee stock ownership plan, employees can accrue company stock in a deferred financial account.
- **Employee stock purchase plan** — Employees can purchase Federal Express common stock at a 15 percent discount rate.

Eastern Air Lines

The Eastern Air Lines-International Association of Machinists' experiment in power sharing began in December, 1983. In the bargain, employees traded wage and productivity concessions for stock and representation on the board of directors. Eastern also granted its unions, most notably the International Association of Machinists, a much larger role in managing the company. Further innovations were negotiated in April, 1985.

Overall the agreement has converted a bitterly confrontational pattern of labor relations into a cooperative one. The new model suggests a marriage of productivity and empowerment. Among the agreements include:

- Eastern gave its employees 25 percent of its common stock (12 million shares) to be held in trust until 1986, plus a new union-preferred security that is convertible to three million shares of Eastern common stock. The stock trust is controlled unilaterally by the union. In effect, labor has three tiers of profit sharing incentives: preferred stock dividends, profit sharing for 1985 of all

net earnings in excess of $90 million, and a dollar-for-dollar productivity buyback of past wage concessions.
- In a power-sharing program, unions have become involved in nearly all aspects of Eastern's management: financial data, corporate planning, routes and fares, and capital investments. The union, on its part, has agreed to a more flexible concept of job assignments, so that traditional work priorities are no longer in the way of the quickest way to complete tasks.
- Under the new employee involvement program, called "Programs for Positive Action," lead mechanics have regained much of their authority to assign work at Eastern. Union crew leaders have now taken responsibility for scheduling and directing work, allowing the company to eliminate an entire tier of supervisors.
- Four board seats were given to workers.

For Eastern, the immediate payoff was a sharp reduction in losses and a return to profitability by the third quarter of 1984. The airline cut operating costs, increased productivity, and set money aside for profit sharing. Formal grievances, which used to exceed 1,000 a year are now running about 400. In-house sources claim that power sharing is now so entrenched in the airline's operations that it is likely to endure. Information sharing has led to something approaching real co-management of the company.

6

Tense Work Relationships

Employees spend over one third of their time at work. Organizational relationships are an influential part of their lives. At work, employees have a strong need to be part of a family and to be a member of a winning team. They thrive on the camaraderie of a high-performing system that also allows them the opportunity to shine on their own. Employees enjoy the comforts of praise, and show time and again that they respond well to positive rewards and healthy work relationships.

For these reasons, relationships at work are one of the strongest determinants of employee health. Healthy companies differ dramatically from unhealthy ones in the quality of their relationships. Healthy companies are open, trusting, predictable, flexible, and supportive. These characteristics apply as much to manager-employee relationships as they do to co-worker and customer relationships. Through these work relationships, healthy companies provide their employees with a sense of belonging and social support, which can buffer the negative effects of stress and protect workers against health breakdowns. This is especially important as other traditional support networks in our society, such as family and church, are breaking down for many people. The absence of such social support leads to feelings of alienation, burnout, and a variety of physical and mental health problems.

Unhealthy companies, in contrast, are mistrustful, unpredictable, and manipulative, and are often characterized by selfish, closed, formal communications. This attitude of mistrust can be caused by numerous factors, sometimes the result of arbitrary policies on the part of management, other times by unhealthy competition among peers. In either case, the workplace turns into a pit of suspicion, hostility, and indifference, imposing unnecessary stress on all those involved.

Unhealthy management values are one form of organizational stress. These values are often unwritten and at times unacknowledged codes of behavior that affect everyone inside a company. Many times these values are reflected in a company's policies and procedures.

For example, the following attitudes and values create work conditions that are stressful and potentially detrimental to one's health.

- "Excessive stress is a mark of excellence."
- "Positive feedback doesn't work as well as punishment."
- "Let's keep our employees guessing."
- "Employees are too naive to participate."

Each of these attitudes can become so ingrained in a corporate culture that their impact is felt at the top of the corporation through management policy and at the bottom via the supervisory process.

Another source of organizational stress is poor supervision, characterized by inconsistency, poor leadership, a lack of concern for the welfare of employees, and constant conflicts with supervisors and subordinates. Bad bosses can make people sick by being unpredictable and setting up win/lose situations, eventually whittling down employee self-esteem. Subordinates working under these managers burn out quickly and experience a variety of health problems.

These types of managers are often undereducated about employee behavior and the impact of their management styles on employee health and productivity. Many are insensitive to the fact that contemporary workers want to be understood and guided, rather than directed and controlled. Others simply lack the skills required to be good managers. Most, unfortunately, do not realize that individual employees are different from one another, and that managing for health and productivity requires a respect for these differences. Some call this "situational management"; others highlight the importance of using the right leadership style in managing for wellness.

Healthy supervisors provide enough information, help, and equipment to get a job done, and give clear responsibilities and enough authority to workers to carry them out satisfactorily. They gain cooperation, provide constructive feedback, recognize the critical importance of reward and reinforcement, and identify employees who are under stress.

Relations with co-workers can be a health risk factor too. For example, ongoing contact with "stress carriers," such as those who either instigate, denegrate, or discourage their fellow employees produces stress for all those around them. Healthy peer competition in a supportive team environment, however, can produce the right amount of stress, just enough to stimulate innovation and productivity without affecting an employee's health.

New office technologies, especially computers, are changing the nature of work relationships. These technologies can create more opportunities for communication and supportive interaction, or they can close off communication and create additional work stress.

For example, the electronic monitoring of an employee's performance at work is now common in many offices. Perhaps surprisingly, this new form of "supervision" can promote health by offering new opportunities for self-management and giving immediate feedback on performance. It can also produce excessive stress by imposing pressure on an employee to produce at a pace established by the machine by taking away employee responsibility when the monitoring occurs and by controlling the way information is used. Perhaps worst of all, it reduces opportunities to interact with others.

Examples of stress sources associated with work relations include:

- Unhealthy management values and policies
- Tense work relationships
- Poor supervision
- Stress-carriers
- Poor communication
- Unhealthy electronic supervision

RESEARCH FINDINGS

Substantial research at the workplace, in the laboratory, and in other settings demonstrates the importance of positive, supportive work relationships as a buffer against the development of stress and disease. Industrial/organizational studies show that poor supervision and inadequate work relations are associated with health problems like coronary heart disease, hypertension, ulcers, alcohol abuse, psychological stress, anxiety and depression, as well as job factors like poor performance and turnover. These studies are consistent with other research that finds the absence of positive social ties a major risk factor for mortality, over and above other known lifestyle risk factors.

Analysis of the famous Framingham heart study data showed that women clerical workers developed coronary heart disease (CHD) at about twice the rate of other women workers and women at home. The workplace factors that most commonly predicted the development of CHD among clerical workers were a nonsupportive boss and low job mobility. Similarly, an Israeli study of 10,000 men 40 years and older found a higher incidence of angina among men who had poor relations with their supervisors. Lack of recognition for a job well done, boredom, and poor relations with co-workers are more often reported by people with coronary heart disease than by those with healthy hearts.

Several other studies have shown that support from supervisors and co-workers is associated with lower levels of work stress and better reports of physical and mental health, while social isolation at work has been shown to be associated with depression, anxiety, job dissatisfaction, muscular fatigue, and psychosomatic symptoms.

Research indicates that certain recurring features in the workplace are responsible for the problem of burnout. Individuals reporting to the same supervisor, for example, are likely to experience similar levels of burnout. This suggests that the policies, practices, and style of the immediate supervisor have a direct bearing on the degree of burnout.

Work units with high levels of burnout have the following profile:

- Low group cohesiveness
- Low supervisory support
- High pressure to produce
- Unclear roles and goals.

CORPORATE APPROACHES

The following is a sampling of a number of corporate programs designed to protect workers against the stressful effects of unhealthy work relationships.

They include:

- Healthy management philosophies and incentives
- Positive organizational health norms
- Supervisory training, coaching, and mentoring program
- Intergroup problem solving, networking, and team building

- Open communication programs
- Recognition/reward programs

A. Healthy Management Philosophies and Incentives

Delta Air Lines, Inc.

Delta's corporate culture is described by its president as an "atmosphere of approval" and a "family feeling." People at all levels of the company are encouraged to work hard, make decisions, speak up if they see areas of concern, and coordinate their ideas and actions with those of other departments. The company claims that this atmosphere creates a spirit of cooperation among departments, places a strong emphasis on learning how Delta approaches problems, and creates a positive place to work.

Leo Burnett Company, Inc.

At Leo Burnett Company, Inc., mistakes are considered part of the business and are incorporated into the firm's organizational health policy. As Burnett himself once said, "The pursuit of excellence is an endless curiosity — searching, throwing away, and trying again . . . a treasure to be nourished and safeguarded. . ." In his Formula for Failure, Burnett observed, "There is no better way to wreck yourself than to seek the security of agreement, by sailing close to the shore, inside the snug harbor of tradition. . . . You will make mistakes, but nobody makes mistakes on purpose. . . . When you do make a mistake . . . you shouldn't let it gnaw at you but should get it out into the open quickly so it can be dealt with; and you'll sleep better too."

Over the years these management philosophies have molded the human resource policies at Burnett. Expressing an alternative point of view, taking chances, and making mistakes are considered part of doing business. At Burnett people have a place to talk and be heard. There is an emphasis on teamwork rather than individual performance, which gives people the freedom to admit mistakes in groups.

There also is an awareness at Burnett that vulnerability and stress are an inevitable part of business. Management gives full support to employees who enter counseling. There are frequent opportunities to change career direction.

B. Positive Organizational Health Norms

Rolm Corporation

Rolm's "Great Place to Work" philosophy:

- Work should be challenging, stimulating, and enjoyable.
- The workplace should be pleasant.
- Every employee should have an opportunity to enhance his or her self-image through achievement, creativity, and constructive feedback.
- Every worker should have equal opportunity to grow and be promoted.
- Every employee should be treated as an individual.
- Personal privacy should be respected.
- Encouragement and assistance to succeed should be provided.
- Opportunities should be available to be creative.
- Evaluation should be based on job performance only.

Hewlett Packard

HP's philosophy (as defined by some managers):

- Belief in people, freedom
- Respect for self-esteem
- Recognition, achievement, and participation
- Employment security and employee development
- Insurance; personal worry protection
- Shared benefits and responsibilities
- Management by objectives rather than by directive
- Decentralization: informality, first names, open communication
- A chance to learn by making mistakes
- Training, education, and counseling
- Performance and enthusiasm

Moog Inc.

Moog believes that by providing an environment of trust and respect, excellent benefits, pleasant surroundings, and security for employees' families, employees will be more committed to the success of the company. Moog demonstrates its commitment to these beliefs through a coordinated set of policies and programs, implemented throughout the company. These include:

- Creating a trusting environment in which there are no time-clocks. Employees report their own time, schedule their own breaks, and inspect their own work. There are no specific rules for personal time off; decisions are made on an individual basis.
- Providing a comfortable, attractive work environment designed to enable most employees, regardless of their location within the plant, to see out a window. Shop floor work is done with benefit of natural light as much as possible and on a white, tile floor kept scrupulously clean by employees.
- Providing special vacation benefits, including a third week of vacation after five years and a seven-week bonus after ten years that can be used either for vacation or taken in cash, with company approval.
- Ensuring the best possible transition into retirement by offering a six-week pre-retirement course for employees and their spouses on legal and health issues of retirement, use of time, financial planning, and other areas of interest to potential retirees.

C. Supervisory Training, Coaching, and Mentoring Program

Northern Telecom, Inc.

Northern Telecom, Inc. recognizes that stress management is good management, and has integrated instruction in individual and organizational stress management into its management training program. The program teaches managers about stress inside and outside the corporation in relation to themselves, their bosses, subordinates, and families. It educates them in stress-reducing techniques, such as good communication, role clarity, predictability, and participative decision-making. Finally, it offers organizational stress seminars to departments as part of departmental team-building.

D. Intergroup Problem Solving, Networking, and Team Building

Xerox

In 1979, Xerox developed a strategy for total employee involvement that projected an evolution from quality circles to full employee participation within ten years. The implementation of this process began in 1980, using the Japanese quality circle concept as a foundation. These developed into a series of problem-solving teams throughout the organization, which over time evolved into what is now know as the "Business Area Work Group" concept.

A business area work group is a cross-functional group with a common output. As many as thirty-five groups consisting of fifteen to fifty employees each blanket an area with 100 percent involvement. Employees meet one and a half hours bi-weekly for communication and problem-solving sessions. Temporary teams are created for specific functions with targeted tasks to perform. The work-group functions emphasize informaion sharing, problem identification, and problem solving. Work group participation is required, but task force participation is optional.

Twenty-four hours of scheduled quality-of-worklife training provides the basic skills needed to become a member of a work group. Employees are able to participate to whatever extent they desire and are taught the skills to do the job effectively. Training is conducted in groups so that team building is emphasized from the outset.

So far, results from the work groups have included:

- Elimination of toxic fumes
- Decreased maintenance material costs
- Decreased clerical paperwork
- Self-managing work teams with control over daily job-related decisions
- Improved ventilation and lighting in service-work areas
- Elimination of unnecessary overhead and reduced downtime for high-volume production machines.

Kollmorgen

Kollmorgen conducts "people meetings" on a regular basis. At these meetings, employees discuss the health of the business, examine whether the company made money, and if not, why not. Managers answer employee questions and concerns, whether raised on the spot or submitted in advance.

The company also conducts "Kolture Sessions" designed to acquaint new employees and reeducate current ones about the Kollmorgen culture and management philosophy. Two-day sessions are held annually involving all levels of employees, including senior management and a mixture of divisions.

TRW

TRW electronics and defense sector regularly uses in-house human resource consultants to develop teams and to facilitate intra- and intergroup problem solving across a wide range of skills and functions. Prior to writing contract proposals, human resource staff help project managers create the right match of personnel for the job in terms of both job skills and personal compatibility.

Human resource staff also perform organizational culture assessments and Quality of Work Life reviews for the various project teams. They circulate throughout a department, interview staff, and assess how well the group is capable of working together and feed back this information to the team members for action and discussion.

At TRW, team building and intergroup problem solving can play an important role in promoting the health of employees. The team concept allows workers who experience stress to talk about it in a relatively open and supportive work environment. When there is increased pressure to produce from colleagues inside the group, sharing solutions and providing social support in a team atmosphere can buffer much of the work stress.

Goldman Sachs & Company

Team performance is critical to success at Goldman Sachs, underscoring the importance of collaborative work relationships. This is becoming more and more important as the company experiences an increasing need for multidisciplinary products and services.

Goldman Sachs recruits bright people who will be good team players; it takes a dim view of internal politics and employees are rewarded for outstanding individual **and** team performance. The emphasis on team building and team performance is pervasive, reinforced by memos from the chairman and supported throughout the supervision and evaluation process.

E. Open Communication Programs

Delta Air Lines

Delta Air Lines believes that open communications are essential to making the best environment for its people. It encourages communication in three ways:

- **Open-Door Policy.** Anyone can go into any office at Delta to voice a problem or complaint.
- **Personnel Rep Program.** All major operating departments have in-house personnel representatives whose jobs are to facilitate communication. All positions are staffed on a rotating basis, and incumbents are selected from the area they represent.
- **Personnel Group Meeting.** Every 18 to 24 months, department heads and personnel representatives host group meetings with their divisions. Current activities of the company, along with a discussion of plans for the future, are discussed. There is also a question and answer period during which all local managers are excused, placing employees in direct contact with their department heads. Response and follow-up are an integral part of these sessions. After each meeting, a summary of the questions is circulated back to the particular station, and a copy is circulated to the division head and chief executive officer.

Hewlett Packard

To ensure open communications at Hewlett Packard, a number of policies and procedures have been instituted, including:

- Informality, such as the use of first names
- No doors on offices
- Network of open partitions
- Permission to learn by making mistakes
- Opportunities to participate and solve problems
- A "Management-by-Wandering-Around" philosophy

Electro Scientific Industries, Inc.

On the assumption that productivity problems are the result of managers getting in the way of employee performance and creativity, ESI operates "Going Well/In the Way" meetings on a regular basis. Small groups of employees (25-30) meet with top-management groups to communicate employee concerns and identify management barriers. Similar communication meetings between departments are used to encourage an open flow of ideas among the technicians, salesforce, business units, and manufacturing divisions.

Cummins Engine Co., Inc.

Cummins Engine believes that the employee's voice is invaluable to its entire operation, and so the company is designed to enable these voices to be heard. There are only two layers between plant workers and the plant manager, and an open-door policy prevails.

Employees function on active decision-making teams. The team manager is responsible for both upward and downward communication, conveying information about business conditions and competition downward to the team and about operating conditions upward to management. Standing representatives and issue committees regularly pass information upward to management about employee dissatisfactions or about operating problems, such as ice in the parking lots or concerns over pay and training.

Cummins feels it makes strong demands on its employees by asking them to "turn their heads on rather than turning their brains off," but it feels that this increased employee participation and the opportunity to communicate has resulted in much higher morale and almost perfect attendence. The company acknowledges, however, that the change in role is sometimes difficult for workers to make, pointing out that "people know when they don't fit." Those few workers generally select themselves out of the company.

F. Recognition/Reward Programs

Holiday Inns

Several hotels in the Holiday Inns chain (Nashville & Knoxville, Tennessee) have instituted a "praising coupon" program which provides guests with a booklet of praising coupons. The guests are instructed to look for employees doing something right and to present that employee with a coupon to be filled out with a description of the positive deed. These coupons are then turned in to the manager, who praises the employee. The response to this program has positively affected absenteeism, morale, and turnover.

7

Lack of Career Progress

In today's workplace employees are moving away from wanting just a nine-to-five job. They now demand that their organizations provide career development and opportunities to develop a variety of skills. Employers are seeing the value in career development as well, especially as technologies change and the need increases for retaining key personnel and competing for talented staff.

Healthy companies are "cultivators of human potential" in which training and development are vehicles for long-term personnel planning. The technical and interpersonal skills of employees are assessed, and succession plans are created to give them a sense of where they stand and how they should move through the organization. Jobs are designed flexibly to meet personal and career objectives, and employees are encouraged to change those aspects of their jobs that are unsatisfying and unhealthy.

Managers are taught to match people to jobs and to reject the "quick fix" approach to stress. They are also sensitive to the career progress of women and minorities. Blocked career paths are avoided whenever possible, and key career transitions, such as promotions, relocations, and transfers, are designed for health and productivity.

Unhealthy companies, in contrast, pay little attention to developing employees. Their focus is short-term, and the concept of "human capital" is ignored. Workers are insufficiently trained and ill-prepared for future markets and jobs within the company. Skills and abilities are poorly monitored and underutilized. Some workers are underpromoted, promoting instead intense feelings of resentment and stress-related illnesses. Others are overpromoted in unfair ways, creating organizational tension. The norm is career stagnation rather than career growth. The desire for recognition, participation, and stimulating work is seldom seen as relevant to bottom line profits. And little attention is paid to matching workers with jobs or supervisors, often creating tense and unproductive work groups.

Examples of stressful career progression include:

- Inadequate career development and growth opportunities
- Insufficient skills or inadequate training
- Underutilization of skills
- Underpromotion/overpromotion
- Unhealthy matches of employees, managers, and jobs

RESEARCH FINDINGS

Several studies have examined the relationship between intrinsic rewards — that is, the chance to develop and use skills, to do interesting work, to learn to believe in what one is doing — and health outcomes. Workers with intrinsically unsatisfying jobs report increased blood pressure, gastrointestinal discomfort, diabetes, cardiovascular risk, and decreased job satisfaction. In jobs where there is little opportunity for promotions, or where promotions are handled unfairly, there is increased antagonism, frustration, depression, and indifference.

A study of middle management executives at Lockheed Corporation found that a poor fit between an employee and his work was related to increasing stress and a higher risk of heart attack based on risk factors such as blood pressure, cholesterol level, adrenalin secretion, and psychological stress. Autonomous, extroverted, achievement-oriented employees were most stressed by work conditions characterized by inadequate freedom to make decisions, excessive guidance and structure, and little personal involvement among workers. Employees who were introverted, humble, and yielding were most stressed by *too much* personal involvement with other workers, too much responsibility for decision making, a crowded work environment, and inadequate guidance from upper management.

Lockheed concluded that a good fit between the worker and his work environment is a responsibility shared by the employee and by the employer. "An enlightened management must appreciate individual differences in employees," the study found, "and improve the quality of worklife by assisting employees in finding a good job fit."

In another study, this one of 2,000 telephone operators, significant differences were noted between those who were chronically sick and those who were relatively free of illness. The two groups differed in how well matched they were in their jobs. Most of the individuals in the chronically sick group had a professional background, with a high school or some college education. They tended to describe their duties as confining or boring, and generally considered themselves frustrated and stuck in wrong jobs. They were unhappy at home as well as at work.

The healthy workers came from lower middle class backgrounds and had an elementary school education. As a group, they appeared to be content with their lives and felt their jobs were satisfying and not overly complex or difficult. These attitudes carried over into a happy home life.

CORPORATE APPROACHES

Following is a sampling of some corporate programs designed to promote health and productivity through various career progression programs. They include:

- Succession planning/matching workers to jobs, teams, and supervisors
- Career development and growth opportunities

A. Succession Planning/Matching Workers to Jobs, Teams, and Supervisors

Exxon

Since 1929, Exxon has felt that identifying and training a successor is the first priority of any manager and an extensive corporate-wide system has been put in place to support this commitment. Each year all positions are examined to identify high-potential people who might best fill future positions in the company. A systematic program of training and development is then set up to help get them there.

Managers throughout the organization review their own positions and the positions of the people reporting to them. For each of these positions, managers determine their subordinates' career potential. Recommendations for filling particular types of positions are circulated world-wide to improve the odds of suitable career advancement and appropriate matching. At the highest level of management, the eight inside directors meet once a week as an executive and compensation committee to examine succession planning and employee development for the 300 positions for which they are responsible.

As part of Exxon's commitment to equal opportunity, all managers are required to review annually the top ten women and minorities in their group, describe what they are doing, and plan for their advancement.

Dayton Hudson

An elaborate succession management planning process is also standard operating procedure at Dayton Hudson. Through a series of interviews and job testing and evaluation, employees' management skills and interpersonal relations are assessed. Dayton Hudson maintains a database on 8,000 salaried people, while at the same time keeping track of job openings inside the company. Job descriptions and "back up" management plans assist in this placement process. The goal is to ensure the best possible match between managers and jobs, and to actively manage their career progression.

McCormick, Inc.

Through the use of "multiple management" committees, McCormick provides a unique opportunity for its employees to serve as "junior" boards of directors. There are fifteen junior advisory boards at McCormick, each comprised of exempt and nonexempt personnel. Typically they serve a six-month term and receive an additional board fee and vacation benefits. Each board decides on its own agenda and projects; each member rates the others' performances on the committee.

Board meetings, which are open to all McCormick personnel, have focused on topics like quality, relocation and transfer policies, and research and development directions and new product development. Recommendations for day-care centers, employee assistance programs, and on-the-job training have been suggested by these boards.

McCormick offers all nonexempt employees open access to jobs through a formal and informal job posting program. Through a formal application process, nonexempt employees are able to bid for any job inside the company. All nonexempt jobs are posted within a commutable regional area and McCormick gives clear preference to exisiting personnel who are qualified for the job. The company encourages employees to circulate as much as possible inside the organization, and promotes the cross pollination of ideas and skills.

B. Career Development and Growth Opportunities

Honeywell, Inc.
(Military Avionics Division)

"A Chance to Grow" is a Honeywell human resource project designed to help supervisors create an environment that will encourage employees to grow both personally and professionally. The project rewards supervisors who provide an environment that encourages personal and professional growth, while giving employees a chance to evaluate their supervisors' skills in providing that environment.

All eligible employees evaluate their supervisors on the following abilities:

- Establishing rapport
- Establishing an understanding of employees' unique characteristics
- Developing a sense of mission
- Developing achievement motivation and a feeling of being valued
- Developing knowledge, skills, and abilities
- Developing supportive team relationships
- Developing independence
- Developing performance excellence
- Developing political savvy

All supervisors responsible for the direction of at least one full-time employee are candidates for an award. Each supervisor whose score is above a certain level receives $200.

Ranier Bancorporation

Ranier Bancorporation offers a unique solution to the concerns of productivity, turnover, and succession planning with an externally designed training program entitled, "Managing Personal Growth (MPG)." Through this program Ranier is able to assist employees in preparing for jobs that meet personal and career objectives.

Designed as a two-day workshop, MPG helps each individual:

- Examine the specific requirements of their jobs
- Identify personal goals, satisfiers, values, talents, limitations, and development needs
- Actively seek the support and feedback of their immediate supervisors

Prior to the workshop, participants and their supervisors assess the relative importance of over 70 process skills to their current job. Participants complete a motivational assessment to identify goals and values that fit their personal definitions of "job satisfaction." They then relate their specific work activities to these values and goals.

A job-focused action plan is designed to increase personal satisfaction by capitalizing on strengths, overcoming deficiencies, and improving on-the-job effectiveness. Ranier reports that the program:

- Boosts motivation, morale, and job satisfaction
- Reduces stress, discontent, and unrealistic job expectations
- Stimulates employees to make better use of their talents

National Aeronautics and Space Administration

NASA's Goddard Space Flight Center initiated its first career development program in 1977. It was targeted at mid-level technical professionals who had plateaued and had few options in the organization. The program was designed to emphasize short-term work assignments as a way for employees to move from their dead-end positions to new growth areas in a trial assignment. Employees were matched to these assignments based on skills, interests and past experience.

Today Goddard offers a variety of services and programs to a wide range of employee groups. It has been designed for employees facing key career transitions, such as moving from clerical support to professional assignments or for technical specialists being moved up to managers or into retirement.

IBM

IBM has introduced "life-span career planning" to help employees manage the inevitability of occupational change. Such planning may encompass multiple career paths, on-the-job development opportunities, career planning workshops, individual career counseling, and mentor-protege relationships.

8

Unclear Work Roles

Organizations are networks of interconnected roles in which employees are asked to perform tasks and take on jobs with their fellow workers. When these tasks and roles are clearly defined, when the rules of the game are clearly stated, employees are generally able to perform their jobs without much difficulty. In healthy companies these expectations are visible for all to see. Employees know what a good job looks like and how their performance will be evaluated.

In unhealthy companies expectations and rewards are unclear, often leading to health and performance problems. Examples might include: (1) jobs where there is confusion about responsibilities; (2) jobs where the goals, expectations, or criteria for evaluation are unclear or unstated; (3) jobs where workers have responsibility for other employees but are not given sufficient authority to manage; and (4) jobs subject to conflicting demands from different supervisors or departments. In each case, the lack of clarity can be frustrating, stressful, and a potential health hazard.

Performance appraisals are one example of a common interaction that can be either health promoting or stress producing. It is through the evaluation process that job roles are defined — or not defined — inside a company.

The health-promoting performance appraisal creates an evaluation climate conducive to learning and growth. By providing managers and employees with an opportunity to match human resource skills with job requirements, one can improve performance and health simultaneously.

In this healthy work environment, employees are evaluated according to their individual needs and job skills, and are recognized and rewarded for their accomplishments — not their personalities. They are given an opportunity to utilize their special abilities and receive appropriate feedback for their work. Employees are told where they stand in the organization and learn about promotional opportunities that lie ahead. Managers clearly identify job objectives for employees, along with the criteria used to measure progress. The healthy performance appraisal encourages rather than discourages ideas, and provides workers with control over their work by offering them the opportunity to obtain feedback about performance at any point.

In contrast, the stress-producing performance appraisal is characterized by inconsistent feedback; unrealistic promotions and rewards; poorly defined job objectives; and little opportunity for employees to identify work stressors or to vent dissatisfactions.

RESEARCH FINDINGS

Unclear goals and job descriptions, conflicting performance demands, and unclear messages from supervisors have been associated with a variety of physical and mental disorders. Research shows that conflicting job demands and conflicts about one's role at work are associated with increases in hypertension, ulcers, abnormal EKG, and tension. Workers also report lower job satisfaction and decreased self-esteem.

Employees who receive unclear messages from their supervisors report increases in physical problems, such as blood pressure, as well as depression. "Boundary employees," defined as those who work inside and outside of their organizations (such as sales personnel and admistrators), frequently feel responsible for and accountable to people and things they cannot control. Disease incidence is significantly higher in people in boundary positions than it is for people whose roles are strictly inside the organization.

CORPORATE APPROACHES

Following is a sampling of some corporate solutions to the problem of job role stress. They include improved job descriptions, flexibility in defining work, individual and group goal-setting programs, performance appraisal, and fair promotion programs, clear rewards, promotions, and disciplinary procedures.

IBM

At IBM, performance planning and setting priorities are considered critical to the development of human resources. One program in particular, the "Performance Planning Process," enlists managers and their subordinates in a collaborative effort to plan and evaluate employee goals. Each employee, together with his or her manager, develops a job description including salary range, job functions, and potential career growth opportunities. A series of jointly developed work objectives are then specified as weekly, near-term (six months, one year) and long-term goals. These work objectives provide a baseline for ongoing performance assessment.

On a daily basis, managers coach employees by helping them reach their specified goals. At IBM, this is considered an important part of the supervisory process. Quarterly reviews are made at the discretion of the manager. All new hires and those who have recently changed jobs receive a formal six month appraisal.

The hope is to give employees a broader view of the organization, its goals, and where their own growth might lead. Opinion surveys are administered in each division every eighteen months to inform top management about employee needs and concerns.

IBM employees always have the opportunity to question the performance planning process. A long-standing open-door policy gives employees the freedom to appeal a decision at any point. Since 1956, the "Speak-Up" program has provided employees with the opportunity to question and complain about any aspect of the IBM experience through a confidential system. Over 15,000 comments are received each year. The informal "Skip-Level Interviewing" process gives employees a chance to talk openly with top executives.

IBM invests $500 million every year on education and training, and much of this is spent on management training. Each "people manager" receives over 40 hours of training per year. Thirty percent of the education during the training period is spent teaching managers about the "performance planning process."

Hoffman La Roche

In a continuing effort to upgrade management skills and promote improvement in job performance, Hoffman La Roche provides managers with a two-day course on managing performance, with additional follow-up consultation services. The course is one in a series of five core required management skills programs for all managers and addresses the following areas of performance management:

- How to plan performance, including a clear statement of performance expectations
- How to monitor employee performance
- How to review performance and conduct a performance review meeting
- How to relate performance to compensation.

The course provides an opportunity for managers to practice key skills in writing job standards/goals, coaching/counseling individual employees, and preparing and delivering a performance review that is videotaped and critiqued. As homework, managers review six months of performance information from a hypothetical employee's monitoring files, and using a review form and some guidelines, prepare notes for the videotaped review session. The following day, managers conduct the reviews with other managers who role play the employee. All participants then review the videotaped sessions, using evaluation forms which examine the content and process used, how the manager draws the employee into the process, handles employee objectives, focuses on areas needing improvement, and creates an employee development plan.

Following completion of the performance management course, managers report greater confidence in conducting performance reviews, and employees report increasingly fair and helpful feedback. The human resource department provides continuing support to managers through follow-up assistance to departments in tailoring and refining performance standards, and training personnel to implement them, as well as assisting individual supervisors in completing and implementing their performance appraisals.

Federal Express

To ensure fair treatment inside the corporation, Federal Express has instituted a five-step complaint process to reduce employee concerns about management and disciplinary decisions. The five-step procedure includes:

1) Frank and informal discussions with supervisors;
2) Discussions with senior manager, director, and vice president-level personnel;

3) Appeal to senior vice president;
4) Optimal Board of Review (employee chooses three of five members and has input into selection of another two);
5) Appeals Board (chairman, chief operating officer, chief personnel officer)

9

Poorly Managed Change

Constant change can be a disruptive form of organizational stress and a potential health hazard for employees. In recent years, much change has been caused by the rapid transition from an industrial, labor-based economy to a technologically advanced, information-based economy, creating new demands along with new forms of work for many employees.

The advent of new technologies has brought with it increased insecurity for workers who fear that their jobs may be phased out. Millions of other workers feel insecurity because of factors such as automation, stricter attendance policies, job reclassifications, or cutbacks. For others, just the threat of unemployment can be devastating to their health and the health of their families.

The use of robotics, for example, has created anxiety for many who don't understand the implication of these new technologies for themselves. The lack of familiarity with computers has similarly made many employees uncertain about their potential impact on their jobs.

Experts have coined the term "technostress" to describe the consequences of this type of automation anxiety. Technostress is a modern disease of adaptation caused by an inability to cope with new computer technologies. It manifests itself in two distinct but related ways: in the struggle to accept computer technology, and in the more specialized form of overidentification with the computer.

Other examples of potentially unhealthy organizational changes include frequent job switches and relocations, rapid alterations in the type of work, poorly managed mergers and acquisitions, and the introduction of new technologies without adequate training.

The historical failure of companies to recognize the devastating effects of such changes, and the failure to build in systematic methods for supporting people through the change process, makes workers feel out of control, helpless, and uncertain about their futures. Poorly managed organizational changes are frequently doomed to failure, as workers either develop debilitating stress symptoms or respond by sabotaging the change process.

Examples of stress associated with technological developments and the change process include:

- Fear of automation and mass technology, such as computer-mediated work, information-processing systems, and robotics
- Inadequate retraining
- Fear of lay-offs or job obsolescence
- Organizational restructing, especially through mergers and acquisitions
- Job shifts and unexplained changes

RESEARCH FINDINGS

Studying the impact of change and new technologies on worker health is a complex task. However, there is research which indicates that poorly managed organizational changes have direct health as well as job productivity consequences. Excessive organizational change has been associated with somatic symptoms, heart disease, anxiety, and decreased job performance. In a ten-year study in Belgium, employees working in a private bank characterized by intense competition and numerous organizational changes had a 50 percent higher incidence of coronary heart disease than those working in a more stable, less pressured public bank.

A study of male workers waiting for the termination of their jobs because of a plant closure found psychological changes in mood and self-identity of the workers. Physiological changes occurred as well, indicating an increased likelihood of coronary disease, diabetes, ulcers, and gout. Data from Johns Hopkins University indicates that every one percent increase in national unemployment is associated with an additional 36,876 deaths, 20,440 from heart disease. There is an attendant increase in alcoholism, crime, family violence, psychological disorders, and hospital admissions. The fear of becoming unemployed places many additional workers and their families at risk of stress disorders.

CORPORATE APPROACHES

Following is a sampling of some corporate programs designed to protect workers against the stressful effects of technology and organizational change. They include:

- Preparing/educating workers about an upcoming change and its implementation process
- Skills training and retooling programs
- Cross training/jobs sharing
- Job security contracts/programs

A. Preparing/Educating Workers About Upcoming Change and Implementation Process

Deere & Company

To ensure that line workers have a full understanding of how new machinery works, Deere sends its employees to the machine's manufacturer. Workers also visit other plants to see how new equipment and procedures are being implemented. Frequently, production workers visit customers and dealers to determine their needs, discuss problems with existing products, and actually operate the equipment in the field. This gives employees a sense of the entire product, from development to customer contact.

Sperry Corporation

To help employees and their families adjust to the relocation of their corporate headquarters from New York City to Blue Bell, Pennsylvania, Sperry Corporation offered two comprehensive assistance programs:

- A special program to encourage and assist workers who accepted offers of transfer. Each employee received:
    — Home-purchase agreement to help with sale of their home.
    — Home-sales incentive bonus.
    — Special orientation to the new community.

- Assistance with new home purchase.
- Pre-move house-hunting trips.
- Interim living expenses following transfer.
- New location allowance equal to one month's pay.
- Moving expenses.
- Transportation of family.
- Special transfer bonus.
- Retirement program vesting.
- Spouse job-seeking assistance.

- A program for those employees who would either not be transferred or who did not feel their personal circumstances would permit them to accept a transfer, including:

  - Income assistance after termination.
  - Supplemental employment bonus during the "phase down" period.
  - 100 percent vesting in the company's retirement program.
  - Continuation of insurance protection for up to six months.
  - Outpatient counseling for employee.
  - Time off for job search.
  - Pay for unused vacation days.
  - Preference for other Sperry employment.

Sperry management realized that office relocation could be a potentially traumatic event for those being transferred, their families, as well as those whose jobs would be terminated. A commitment to equity and credibility would be necessary to buffer this transition. At Sperry, all employees were informed immediately following the relocation decision by top management.

B. Skills Training and Retooling Programs

General Motors

Beginning in 1982, and renegotiated in 1984, General Motors and the United Auto Workers combined forces to develop an extensive skill development and training program for active employees and employees on layoff. Two separate programs were implemented: one to retrain and place laid-off workers, and a second to upgrade the skills of the workforce.

The first program, financed by a contribution of five cents an hour per UAW employee, funded a human resource center where laid-off GM/UAW workers could be retrained, counseled, and placed into new jobs. Approximately $40 million annually is earmarked for this program.

A second program, implemented in five regional training centers, was more preventive in nature, upgrading the existing skills of employees to ensure that their skills remained current with changing technologies. This program is funded through another contribution of ten cents an hour per UAW member.

Communications Workers of America

The Communications Workers of America's (CWA) 1980 contract with AT&T established a joint Quality of Work Life (QWL) process. In their 1983 national contract, union and management reaffirmed their commitment to this process. Local QWL teams have solved a range of workplace problems and, in a few cases, have formed semi-autonomous work groups.

As a part of their 1983 contract, CWA and AT&T also agreed to training provisions. As called for in the contract, joint union-management Training Advisory Boards were created with AT&T and each of the local Bell Operating Companies. The contract directed each company to offer free training outside of working hours to help potentially displaced workers retrain for new jobs within the company and other workers qualify for promotions.

On January 1, 1984, AT&T was divested of the Bell Operating Companies (BOCs). CWAs 1983 contract provisions on QWL and training now applied separately to AT&T and the independent BOCs. Today, there are about 3,000 local QWL committees, and surveys in some companies show increased worker satisfaction. In addition, AT&T and most of the BOCs have offered free, off-hours training under the guidance of the joint Training Advisory Boards.

C. Cross Training/Job Sharing

Nissan Motor Manufacturing Company, USA

Nissan's cross training and "Pay for Versatility" programs provide employees with financial compensation for broadening their work skills.

In the cross-training program, assembly-line workers are taught a variety of jobs and skills. Each employee is required to learn each job in his supervisor's "zone." Workers rotate jobs every few hours, especially in jobs that are repetitious. Nissan reports that the program boosts morale, reduces stressful, monotonous work, and decreases the frequency of wrist, shoulder, and lower back ailments.

The "Pay for Versatility" program supports cross-training by linking skill development to financial compensation. All manufacturing employees are eligible for the program after three years or following a transfer to another department. Cross training is made available across a number of skill areas. If an employee participates, he receives a bonus of 25 cents an hour for production workers and 30 cents an hour for maintenance workers. The bonus is retained if the worker remains open to cross-training opportunities. Nissan reports that employee skills are constantly evolving, reducing the threat of job obsolescence.

Motorola

In an attempt to both deal effectively with periodic downturns in the electronics industry and also to deal fairly with employees, Motorola has supported a new approach to job sharing to avoid large-scale layoffs in its industry. This voluntary program, begun in California, is called "shared work unemployment compensation."

Through a cooperative arrangement with the state unemployment agency, California corporations can identify groups of workers and reduce their work hours up to 40 percent, while having those lost hours covered by unemployment compensation. Using this program, Motorola has been able to weather downturns in the industry by using stable, seasoned workers and avoiding costly rehiring and training. The company was able to reduce the hours of 9,000 employees by 10 percent to save $3 million; Under a similar plan in Arizona, the company estimates savings of $1,800 per employee. In each case, employees have been guaranteed continued employment and benefits while receiving at least 85 percent of their normal salary. Motorola has lobbied successfully in nine states to create similar programs.

D. Job Security Contracts/Programs

Delta Air Lines, Inc.

Delta's long-standing policy of promoting from within the company in filling supervisory, management, and higher level administrative and staff functions is considered vital to the success of the organization. Over the years Delta has also avoided using involuntary furloughs to cut labor costs, and has striven to hold to this policy even when downturns in business left the company temporarily overstaffed. Delta believes that although its competitors may gain short-run advantages, the consistency of its promotion and layoff policies wins the long-range battle with higher morale and greater productivity.

An additional benefit is that individuals in the organization know they have job security and an opportunity for advancement. They are not competing with unknown individuals from outside the company. Over time, employees get to know the business and management gets to know its people.

Promotion from within places a heavy responsibility on the initial employment function. Those who join Delta must be willing to commit themselves to the organization, and must be capable of growing and undertaking more tasks and duties.

Hallmark Cards

Rather than terminating employees, Hallmark Cards has a commitment to solve staffing and downsizing problems inside the corporation. Designed as a "no layoff practice," the corporation employs several strategies:
- Use of voluntary time off without pay whenever possible.
- Filling vacancies from within.
- Moving people around inside the company in temporary departmental transfers.

Advanced Micro Devices

AMD's policies for dealing with the recent 30 to 40 percent volume reductions in its semiconductor market reflect its attitude of "People first; products and profits will follow." Currently, as the only semiconductor firm in Silicon Valley with an active "no layoff policy," AMD continues to cope by taking actions that maintain its commitment to employees. AMD believes that if people are to be loyal and dedicated, they must be treated fairly. The company has instituted several actions to reach this goal:

- 10 percent pay cuts for all exempt employees.
- 15 percent cuts for all executive staff.
- Deferred raises.
- Two-week shutdown over Christmas, during which time employees in applicable states may use job-sharing benefits in conjunction with state unemployment agencies.

AMD feels these programs have enabled it to maintain high morale. Evidence of this is a turnover rate of only 12 to 14 percent for exempt personnel despite the short-term costs of keeping them on.

Hewlett Packard

To protect workers against the negative effects of changing technology, Hewlett Packard has instituted the following policies:

- No layoffs.
- Retrain employees with obsolescent skills, and redirect employees into new areas of business.
- Promotion from within the company.
- Develop a "resource referral" network inside the company.
- Be open to alternative work schedules. For example, to protect the company against the temporary flattening of the computer market, in July, 1985 most HP employees (with the exception of field sales people) took two days a month without pay. The policy was temporary. As the company improves, HP will resume its original schedule.

10

Work/Family/Leisure Conflicts

In recent times, job demands have competed head on with other interests and responsibilities outside of work, such as family, education, leisure, and avocational interests. Many workers now pursue several careers in a lifetime, and are involved in numerous hobbies and educational activities outside the workplace. Employees are striving to improve their "quality of life," yet feel pressured by a lack of time to accomplish both work and nonwork activities. Job demands and leisure interests compete for limited time, potentially resulting in unhealthy stress and productivity problems.

Work and leisure conflicts are particulary manifest in family life. With increasing numbers of working women and two-career families, many parents must balance career pursuits, child rearing, and an intimate relationship simultaneously. The problems of single-parent families are even more pronounced. Aging parents, young children, family illness, and work deadlines also compete for attention. The health and performance effects of these conflicting work and family roles can be overwhelming.

The transition from worklife into retirement is another example of the work-leisure dilemma. As our population ages, and as new technologies demand new kinds of work skills, many employees are confronting job obsolescence and forced retirement prematurely. These conditions are slowly forcing companies to re-examine their retirement policies and programs, particularly as they affect the health and performance of their workforce.

At this point little is known about the impact of these changing conditions on employee health and the bottom line. Unfortunately, most corporations have overlooked how family and leisure conflicts affect their bottom lines, and continue to design policies that meet the needs of the traditional working male breadwinner and his homebound wife, rather than meeting the needs of the new work and family roles.

WORK AND FAMILY STRESS

The following statistics highlight the seriousness of the growing health and productivity problems associated with work and family conflicts.

Dramatic Increase in Number of Working Women and Working Mothers

Today, women make up more than 40 percent of the workforce, a three-fold increase since 1940. During the same period, the number of working mothers has gone up ten times. In 1982, almost 60 percent of the mothers of children under 18 were working.

Women Return to Work Sooner after Pregnancy

In 1983, 30 percent of children were born to mothers who worked during their pregnancy — a number expected to rise. It is estimated that by 1990, 80 percent of working women will be raising babies at some period during their work lives. On average, women now return from maternity leave within four months after giving birth, and approximately one-third of mothers with babies under six months are working.

Insufficient Child Care Services Limit Adequate Supervision

Nearly half of all children under six have working mothers. In 1981, 45 percent of the 8.2 million pre-school children had mothers who were in the workforce. Unfortunately, there was only enough licensed child care to serve 25 percent of these children. Only 1.7 million of the over 30 million school-age children whose mothers worked participated in an organized before- or after-school child care programs. The U.S. Bureau of the Census now estimates that approximately two million youngsters between ages seven and 13 are routinely without adult supervision for some periods of the day.

Rise in Single-Parent Families

More than 12 million children — one of every five in the U.S. — live with single mothers who are the sole breadwinners in their households.

The message from these statistics is clear: women are entering the workforce at an accelerated pace, and most are raising children — infants, toddlers, and school-age — while they work. Many are married, but an increasing number are not. The impact of these conditions on family health and work performance are costly in terms of increased absenteeism, turnover, and stress-related ailments, making this issue a major business and public health problem.

RESEARCH FINDINGS

Only a limited number of studies have looked explicitly at how work and non-work demands combine to influence health and productivity. Even fewer studies have focused specifically on the work and family conflict.

Studies of working women sometimes find poorer health among those who also have significant child-rearing responsibilities. Working women of child bearing age are absent from their jobs more than they should be.

When Honeywell, Inc., surveyed its employees in 1980, it found that one of four working parents believed that stress caused by child care problems interfered with their productivity and caused high absenteeism. At Control Data Corporation headquarters in Minneapolis, employee parents who enrolled their children in the consortium day care center, which the company helps support, reduced their absenteeism by 21.4 percent compared to their pre-enrollment record. The turnover rate is 2.3 percent per month among center users versus 6.2 percent for those who do not use it.

A study at Texas Women's University showed that a $50,000 investment in a day-care program can save some $3 million in employee turnover, training, and lost work time, much of which is health-related. And a national study recently conducted by the Child Care Information

Service of Pasadena, California, surveyed 415 employers who provide some form of assistance to their employees who must use child care. According to the employers, providing child care assistance was a positive factor in the following ways: attracting employees, lowering absenteeism and job turnover rates, increasing productivity, and improving employee morale.

A Stanford University survey quizzed employees about the advantages of job sharing, and found that the energy and efficiency of employees was increased; there was renewed spirit and motivation; there was less stress because they were able to share their burden with someone else; employers could obtain a better range of skills than might be found in a single individual; and employers could take advantage of the unique contribution of each person.

Interestingly, one study found that people on flextime spent an additional hour with their families.

CORPORATE APPROACHES

Employers are addressing the needs of working parents in a variety of ways, which fall into three categories: (1) providing information about work and family issues (for example, information to help parents locate day care); (2) providing or subsidizing child care (such as financial assistance, vouchers, in-kind services, child care centers); and (3) adjusting personnel policies and work options to accommodate families (including flextime, job sharing/part-time, maternity and paternity leave, sick days for child care).

Information-Based Programs

Aetna Life & Casualty Company

The Aetna Institute for Corporate Education at Aetna Life and Casualty Company sponsors a family and work course for employees, who can receive prepaid college credits at the University of Connecticut. The objective of the course is to facilitate the participants' ability to entertain both family members' and co-workers' viewpoints. The curriculum includes topics on family and work in other cultures, the socialization of work at home, realizing equality at home and at work, new work options, employee benefits and responsibilities, health-care cost management, stress management, child and parent care, promotion, transfer, plateauing, and retirement options.

CBS, Inc.

At CBS, it was found that employees were extremely interested in their children's development and wanted to know how they could enhance it within the time they have with their children. Parents' groups were organized according to the ages of their children:infants/toddlers, preschoolers, school age, and adolescents. Attendance was limited to 25 per session. Parents were able to discuss their specific concerns, from toilet training to activities for adolescents.

Honeywell, Inc.

Honeywell donated $25,000 and staff time to help three day-care agencies develop a computerized child care information network. The service collects, updates, and exchanges data on child care programs. Honeywell also has a working-parent resource coordinator who shapes policy and acts as liaison between parent-employees, their supervisors, educators in the community, and representatives of outside companies.

IBM

IBM has sponsored the development of information and referral services throughout the country to serve its 218,000 employees in over 200 cities. Employees receive information and counseling about child care.

Hartford Corporate Consortium

A child care information and referral program was created by a consortium of companies in Hartford, Connecticut. The program has access to licensed child care programs in 38 towns and cities in the Hartford area. Some of the participating companies include the Travelers Insurance Company, Connecticut Bank & Trust Company, the Connecticut National Bank, Hartford Steam Boiler Inspection, and Aetna Life and Casualty.

Providing/Subsidizing Child Care

Nyloncraft, Inc.

The Nyloncraft Learning Center and Child Care Service was initiated by management of Nyloncraft, Inc. The primary impetus was management's concern for working parents, and the need to reduce their excessive absenteeism and turnover. The company provided funding for the design, construction, and equipment of the center. Nyloncraft also subsidizes the cost of child care for its employees' children. The goals of the center are to:

- Provide a quality child development/daycare program.
- Provide a model for employer-supported child care.
- Serve the needs of working parents.
- Provide needed child care services to the community.

Benefits to parents and children include:

- Child care tax credit.
- Reduced anxiety through reliable and affordable child care.
- Proximity to children, especially in case of emergency.
- An educational program for children.
- Health screening and nutritious meals.

Benefits to Nyloncraft:

- Tax credits.
- Reduced turnover.
- Reduced absenteeism.
- A retention and recruitment tool.
- Positive public relations.
- Increased employee morale.

The Nyloncraft Learning Center is a 24-hour facility, open to community families and licensed by the State Department of Public Welfare. It is designed for working parents with various work schedules and offers educational programs to children from ages 24 months to 13 years. The staff-to-child ratio at the center is 1:18.

In 1979, Nyloncraft had a 57 percent turnover rate. By 1983, that rate had dropped to 9 percent. The company reports that a combination of economic factors, a union contract, and the learning center were responsible for that reduction.

Wang Labs

As a company with many highly skilled women, Wang Labs became concerned about the special needs of working parents, and decided to study the issue of child care. After surveying the need, Wang determined that it would serve its workforce and the community by establishing a child care center. The center is open between 6:30 am to 6:00 pm each day. The company subsidizes employee costs. Wang also purchased a nearby country-club for use as a summer camp for its employees' school-age children.

Baxter Travenol

Baxter subsidizes child care for all corporate headquarters staff at two local centers, providing one-third of the tuition. The program is used by about 10 percent of the staff. Returning employees often cite the program as a major reason for rejoining Baxter-Travenol.

Corning Glass

As a joint venture of the Corning Glass Work Foundation and the community, a daycare center was established and housed in the First Presbyterian Church in Corning, New York. A task force study of the needs of 8,000 parents in Corning was first conducted to determine the need for a center. The foundation provided a grant for the start-up of the center, and additional monies for an information and referral service.

Half of the center's children have parents who are Corning employees and the other half are from the community. The board of directors consists of Corning management personnel, parents, and residents.

CHANGING PERSONNEL POLICIES/WORK OPTIONS

Hewlett Packard

Consistent with Hewlett Packard's philosophy that individuals are responsible for their own development and performance, the company gives employees the freedom to control their own time. Employees can work any eight-hour period during their shift with the approval of their supervisors. There are no time clocks.

A "Flexible Time Off" policy gives workers maximum freedom to control their own off-work time. There is no specific amount of time allocated to sick leave or vacation. Rather, employees are given a set number of personal days to be managed by the individual employee. The practice is one way of acknowledging the tremendous diversity in workers' lifestyles.

Rolm Corporation

To avoid the stress of heavy rush hour traffic and to accommodate employees' personal needs for such things as child rearing and extra curricular activities, Rolm provides workers with opportunities to schedule their own work hours. Each employee negotiates a contract with his/her individual manager.

Time, Inc.

To assist in managing work and family responsibilities, Time, Inc. offers its employees a parental leave of up to one year. The exact job cannot be guaranteed on return to the company, but Time does try to provide a comparable job, assuming one exists. All benefits are maintained throughout the leave period.

Employees who are not placed in a job upon return are eligible for notice and severance.

In addition to these examples, employers as diverse as Levi Strauss & Company, Rolscreen Company, Pan American World Airways, and Kettering Medical Center have instituted "job sharing" arrangements to enhance flexibility for employees and employers, and to reduce stress for workers and their families.

11

Retirement

The transition from older worker to retiree presents a unique set of challenges and opportunities for employees, their families, and their employers. Many employees approach this time with a healthy, positive view, finding new opportunities and exploring alternative hobbies and new relationships.

Many others, however, struggle through the transition, letting the change chisel away at their health and productivity. Most companies respond in a similar fashion, overlooking the issue altogether and rarely examining how retirement affects employee health or their bottom line.

Fortunately, some employers are now realizing the importance of managing employee retirement as they would any other human resource issue. Two approaches shown to have positive effects on health and productivity are retirement transition programs and retraining and education.

Retirement Transition Programs

To help older workers prepare for retirement, some companies have begun offering alternative work arrangements. These can include either restructured full-time work or reduced work arrangements. Examples of restructured full-time work include flextime, a compressed work week, and work-at-home. Examples of reduced-work arrangements include phased retirement, job sharing, work sharing, permanent part-time work, and leaves of absence.

Polaroid

The Polaroid Company offers "retirement rehearsals." These are leaves of absence that allow employees to see what retirement is like, with the option of rejoining the workforce at the end of the leave. It also offers a tapering-off period during which the employee can reduce the number of hours worked per week as a transition to retirement.

Aerospace Corporation

The Aerospace Corporation offers its employees three retirement transition plans: part-time work for less than 20 hours per week, a reduced workload at 20-40 hours per week, and unpaid leaves of absence.

Travelers Insurance

Travelers Insurance Company of Hartford has developed the "Travelers Program for Older Americans," which is based on the belief that business can play a significant role in shaping the future progress of older Americans through activities in the workplace, the marketplace, and the community. In the workplace there is elimination of mandatory retirement, availability of temporary and part-time positions for retirees, a retiree job bank, a pension policy allowing retirees to work nearly half-time without loss of retirement income, and a retirement planning program.

Bankers Life/Chevron

A number of firms, such as Bankers Life and Casualty Company of Chicago and the Chevron Corporation in California, offer comprehensive pre-retirement planning programs to help older workers better understand their options.

Tektronix

Tektronix in Oregon allows individuals to retire and then return to work at the firm, typically in more flexible work environments, if they find retirement unsatisfactory.

ARCO

The Atlantic Richfield Company provides its former employees with a retirement handbook, a special retiree edition of the company newsletter, a toll-free retiree hotline, and retiree clubs as part of its retiree transition program.

Commercial State Bank

Commercial State Bank of St. Paul has a special program offering retirees part-time work as messengers, parking attendants, and clerks.

Woodward and Lothrop

Woodward and Lothrop, a Washington, D.C. retail chain, has a program of flexible work hours for older workers.

R.H. Macy

R.H. Macy, the New York retail chain, offers transitional work schedules to individuals to help them prepare for retirement.

Northern Natural Gas Company

Northern Natural Gas Company has developed job-sharing options that provide reduced work schedules for older workers, enabling them to provide on-the-job training to younger, less experienced workers with whom they share jobs.

Levi-Strauss

Levi-Strauss has a job-sharing program that assists both older and younger employees in sharing a single full-time position.

Retraining and Education Programs

To help older workers keep their skills current in a changing economy, companies are offering a variety of education and retraining programs.

Bank of America

The Bank of America's redeployment policy helps make optimum use of employees' skills, knowledge, and abilities while helping the bank rebalance its work force to meet the demands of technological change and deregulation. Through redeployment, employees whose jobs have been eliminated may opt for an internal search for another assignment or may elect to resign. Workers may also undergo retraining, partially funded by industry-government partnerships, to help them meet the skill requirements of new jobs.

AT&T/Communication Workers of America

AT&T and the Communications Workers of America have negotiated a new labor agreement that calls for the company to provide retraining to workers affected by technological change, many of whom are older workers.

General Motors/United Auto Workers

In its most recent contract with the UAW, General Motors established a job bank for workers laid-off by new technology, productivity improvements, and so forth. These workers are to be retrained for new jobs, either inside or outside General Motors. The company also established a new ventures fund to help develop and launch new businesses that would employ displaced auto workers, many of whom are older. GM expects some of these new ventures to become suppliers to the auto industry.

Ford Motor Company

Ford Motor Company, as part of its 1982 UAW contract, agreed to a guaranteed income stream benefit program for laid-off high-seniority (generally older) workers.

Intertek

Intertek of Los Angeles provides lists of retirees with experience in quality control and inspection to over 200 corporations nationwide.

McDonald's

McDonald's Corporation contracts with local agencies to recruit and place older workers.

Lockheed

Lockheed and other aerospace companies rehire retirees to fill crucial positions in engineering and skilled machine operations.

ARCO/Levi Strauss

The Atlantic Richfield Company and Levi Strauss support a program at the Andrus Gerontology Center of the University of Southern California to help make managers more sensitive to older employees in the workforce.

Operation ABLE

Operation ABLE (Ability Based on Long Experience) is a Chicago-based not-for-profit organization dedicated to promoting employment opportunities to mature adults by offering employers a free source for professional, clerical, and service employees for full-time, part-time, and temporary work; and by offering seekers support training, job search assistance (for professional, managerial, technical, and skilled clerical employees) and an outplacement program. Operation ABLE was founded in 1977 and is supported through grants from public and private sectors, including over 45 major corporations and foundations.

Appendix

The following is a list of some of the companies where an identified program is viewed as contributing significantly to corporate health. We have also provided names of contacts at these organizations.

Advanced Micro Devices
901 Thompson Place
Sunnyvale, CA 94088
Steve Strain, Director, Human Resources
(408) 732-2400 or 749-2094

Argonne National Laboratories
9700 Cass Avenue, Building 202
Argonne, IL 60439
Charles Ehret, Senior Scientist
(312) 977-3862

Baxter Travenol
Travenol Laboratories
1 Baxter Parkway
Deerfield, IL 60015
Jackie Barry, Supervisor of Employee Services

Corning Glass Works
Houghton Park
Corning, NY 14830
Susan King, Vice President & Director of Corporate Communications
(607) 974-9000

Cummins Engine Co., Inc.
605 Cottage Avenue
Columbus, IN 47201

Healthy Companies—103

Richard Christiansen/Joseph Pegahoff — Jamestown
(812) 377-5000

Dana Corporation
P.O. Box 1000
Toledo, OH 43679
Don Decker, Director, Public Relations
(419) 535-4601

Dayton Hudson
777 Nicollet Mall
Minneapolis, MN 55402
Ed Wingate, Senior Vice President, Human Resource Development
(612) 370-6948

Deere & Company
John Deere Road
Moline, IL 61265
James V. Gayle, Manager, Employee Participation
(309) 752-4061

Delta Airlines, Inc.
Hartsfield Atlanta International Airport
Atlanta, GA 30320
Jackie Pate, Manager, Public Relations
(704) 765-2342

Donnelly Corporation
414 East 40th Street
Holland, MI 49423
Bill Lalley
(616) 394-2444

DuPont
1007 Market Street
Wilmington, DE 19898
J.H. Todd, Director, Safety and Occupational Health
(302) 773-4190

Eastman Kodak Company
343 State Street
Rochester, NY 14650
Bill Golden, Manager, Suggestion Program
(716) 724-7264

Electro Scientific Industries, Inc.
13900 N.W. Science Park Drive
Portland, OR 97229

Beverly Lutx, Director of Human Resources
(503) 641-4141

Erie Family Life Insurance Co.
144 E. 6th Street
Erie, PA 16530
Keith Lane, Communications
(814) 452-6831

Exxon
1251 Avenue of the Americas
New York, NY 10020
Woodie Maden, Human Resources Development Department
(212) 333-1000

Exxon Chemical Americas
13501 Katy Freeway
Houston, Texas 77079-1398
Susan Szita Gore, Public Relations Manager
(713) 870-6000

Federal Express
4009 Airways Boulevard
Memphis, TN 38116
Walter Duhaine, Senior Manager, Employee Benefits
(901) 922-5450

Federal Express
P.O. Box 727
Memphis, TN 38196
Andrew Rogers, Manager of Employee Relations
(901) 922-3519

Fisher Price
636 Girard East
Aurora, NY 14052
Mary Ann Lambertson
(716) 687-3447

H.B. Fuller
1200 West County Road East
St. Paul, MN 55112
Mary Marshall
(612) 481-4606

General Motors/United Auto Workers
GM Building, Room 11-211
3044 W. Grand Blvd.

Detroit, MI 48202
John Grix
(313) 492-7128

Goldman Sachs & Company
85 Broad Street
New York, NY 10004
John Weinberg, Managing Partner
(212) 902-1000

Hallmark Cards
P.O. Box 580
Kansas City, MO 64141
Charlie Hucker, Division Vice President of Corporate Communications
(816) 274-5522

Hewlett Packard
3000 Hanover, MS 20 AR
Palo Alto, CA 94304
Frank Williams, Manager of Communication
(415) 857-8425

Hewlett Packard
3000 Hanover Street
Palo Alto, CA 94304
Art Dauer, Director, Human Resources
(415) 857-1501

Honeywell, Inc.
9900 Brent Road East
Suite 420
Minnetonka, MN 55343
James Widfeldt, Associate Director, Quality Management Systems
(612) 931-7593

IBM
Old Orchard Road
Armonk, NY 10504
Roy Westmoreland
(914) 765-5628

Hoffman La Roche
340 Kingsland Street
Nutley, NJ 07110
Carol Brand, Associate Director,
Management and Organizational Development
(201) 235-5050

McCormick, Inc.
11350 McCormick Road

Hunt Valley, MD 21031
Nick Simon, Director of Management Training and Development
(301) 667-7609

Merrill Lynch
165 Broadway, 29th floor
New York, NY 10080
Linda Pattari, Vice President, Management Resources
(212) 637-5159

Herman Miller, Inc.
8500 Byron Road
Zeeland, MI 49464
J. Douglas Zimmerman, Director
Facilities Management Operations
(616) 772-5130

Moog, Inc.
East Aurora, NY 14052
Joyce Fleischer
(716) 652-2000

Motorola
1776 K Street, N.W., Suite 300
Washington, D.C. 20006
Lou Hastings
(202) 862-1500

Nissan Motor Manufacturing Company, USA
Nissan Drive
Smyrna, TN 37167
Hugh Harris, Director of Personnel Relations
(615) 355-2200

Northern Telecom
200 Athlem Way
Nashville, TN 37228
Jeff Harris, M.D., Director, Health & Safety
(615) 734-4952

Northwestern Mutual Life Insurance Company
720 E. Wisconsin Avenue
Milwaukee, WI 53202
Robert W. Ninneman, Senior Vice President, Operations
(414) 271-1444

Nyloncraft, Inc.
Valley Plaza Complex, Suite 8
2410 Grape Road
Mishawaka, IN 46544
(219) 255-3143

Ranier Bancorporation
P.O. Box 3966 N. 05-5
Seattle, WA 98124
Linda Lewis, Vice President, Manpower Development
(206) 621-4138

Rolm Corporation
4855 Patrick Henry Drive, Mailstop 605
Santa Clara, CA 95054
Ken Rowe, Director, Public Relations
(408) 986-5674

Sperry Corporation
1290 Avenue of the Americas
New York, NY 10104
Michael R. Losey, Staff Vice President, Personnel Relations
(212) 484-4642

3M Company
3M Center, 220-13-N
St. Paul, MN 55144
Christopher Wheeler, Executive Vice President, Human Resources
(612) 733-0592

Time, Inc.
1271 6th Avenue
New York, NY 10020
Judith Pinto, Associate Director, Management Resources
(212) 586-1212

TRW
Electonics and Defense Division, One Space Park E2-4000
Redondo Beach, CA 90278
Tom Wickes, Vice President, Employee Relations
(213) 535-1501

Wang Labs
1 Industrial Ave.
Lowell, MA 01851
Paul Guzzi, Vice President, Public Relations
(617) 841-4111

Xerox
North American Manufacturing Division
800 Phillips Road, Bldg. 205-99E
Webster, NY 14580
Larry Pace, Manager
Employee Involvement and Organizational Effectiveness
(716) 422-6646